An Hachette UK Company
www.hachette.co.uk

First published in Great Britain in 2018 by Aster, an imprint of
Octopus Publishing Group Ltd, Carmelite House,
50 Victoria Embankment, London EC4Y 0DZ
www.octopus.co.uk

Distributed in the US by Hachette Book Group, 1290 Avenue of the
Americas, 4th and 5th Floors, New York, NY 10104

Distributed in Canada by Canadian Manda Group, 664 Annette St.,
Toronto, Ontario, Canada M6S 2C8

ISBN 978-1-91202-377-6

A CIP catalogue record for this book is available from the
British Library.

Printed and bound in China.

10 9 8 7 6 5 4 3 2 1

Consultant Publisher Kate Adams
Recipe Developer and Food Stylist Nicole Pisani, Food for Happiness
Senior Designer Jaz Bahra
Assistant Editor Nell Warner
Copy Editor Clare Sayer
Photographer Issy Croker
Food and Props Stylist Emily Ezekiel
Production Manager Caroline Alberti

Picture credits: 7 Quagga Media/Alamy Stock Photo; 9 pierivb/iStock;
11 Science History Images/Alamy Stock Photo; 16-17 renacall/iStock

THE
CACAO
COOKBOOK

Discover the health benefits
and uses of cacao, with
50 delicious recipes

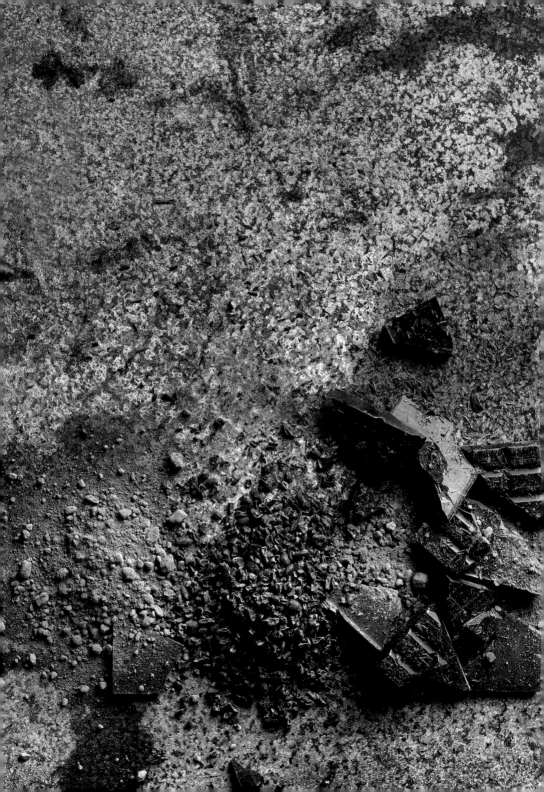

CONTENTS

INTRODUCTION 6
CACAO TRADITIONS 10
THE CACAO CEREMONY 12
THE HEALTH BENEFITS OF CACAO 14
COOKING WITH CACAO 18
BEVERAGES 20
BREAKFASTS 30
SOUPS & SIDES 50
MAIN DISHES 66
SWEETS 92
BEAUTY 116
INDEX 126

INTRODUCTION

Cacao, or *Theobroma cacao* (Greek for "food of the gods"), is the source of original, natural chocolate. Cacao as an ingredient comes from the seeds of the fruit of the cacao tree and has been revered by the indigenous peoples of South America, or Mesoamerica (which includes Mexico, Central America, and South America) as far back as 1600 BC.

Before cacao was cultivated as a crop, it was used in rituals, including religious ceremonies, births, marriages, and funerals, and as a medicine. As it became a type of currency, cacao began to be cultivated, especially by the Mayans around AD 600.

Columbus was the first European to come across cacao in 1502, and a couple of decades after this initial discovery, Cortez then recorded the use of cacao in the court of Emperor Montezuma.

It would be 1657 before the first hot chocolate shop was opened in London, and in the United States, Baker's Chocolate was founded in 1780, producers of the type of chocolate we are familiar with today.

There are three main varieties of cocoa bean used in the production of chocolate or cacao products.

Forastero

This high-yield variety of the cacao tree represents the majority of the world's total cocoa production. *Forastero* means "stranger" or "outsider" in Spanish. It is found in Ghana, Nigeria, Ivory Coast, New Guinea, Brazil, Central America, Sri Lanka, Malaysia, and Indonesia.

Criollo

This is a higher quality and less bitter cocoa bean than forastero, so it tends to be used to make higher quality chocolate. This explains why single-origin chocolate produced from criollo beans is so desirable (and expensive), especially because it is also relatively rare. It is found in Venezuela, Mexico, Nicaragua, Guatemala, Colombia, Samoan Islands, Sri Lanka, and Madagascar.

Trinitario

Forastero beans were cross-fertilized with criollo beans in Trinidad after a hurricane in 1727 destroyed the plantations. These are, therefore, found mainly in the Caribbean, but they can also be found in Venezuela and Colombia.

The large football-like pods that grow on cacao trees are harvested and cracked open to release the cacao beans. The beans are covered with banana leaves and placed in a type of wooden bin or pit in the ground to ferment. This begins the transformation of the beans from their extremely bitter natural state into the main ingredient for chocolate. After fermentation, the beans are dried in the sun before being transported to the manufacturer for processing.

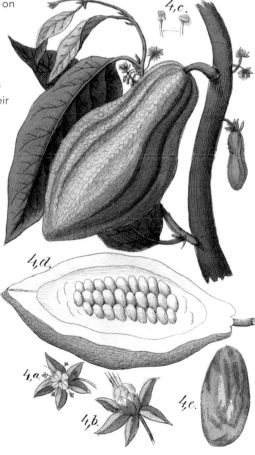

Right: Theobroma Cacao

Cacao versus cocoa

Cacao and cocoa both come from the cocoa bean, the difference is in the amount of processing. Cacao is made by cold-pressing unroasted cacao beans, whereas cocoa is raw cacao that has been roasted at high temperatures; it is then usually sweetened with sugar. Cocoa still has many of the nutrients that cacao has (*see* page 14–15), just in smaller quantities due to the heat in the processing.

The different types of cacao

Once cacao beans are dried, they are cold-pressed to remove the cacao butter, the fatty part of the fruit found in the inner part of the lining of the bean. The beans are then either ground to create raw cacao powder or crushed to create the nibs. Solid cacao is a combination of the raw cacao powder and cacao butter:

- **Cacao powder** has a bitter chocolaty taste.
- **Cacao nibs** are similar to chocolate chips but are more bitter and "savory" in taste.
- **Solid (100 percent) cacao chocolate** is an extremely dark, especially bitter chocolate with no sugar added, made by combining raw cacao powder and cacao butter.
- **Cacao butter** is white in color and buttery and chocolaty in texture; it has an incredible aroma of chocolate. It's used to make chocolate and natural beauty products (*see* pages 96 and 116–125).

Opposite: Cacoa pods from Madagascar

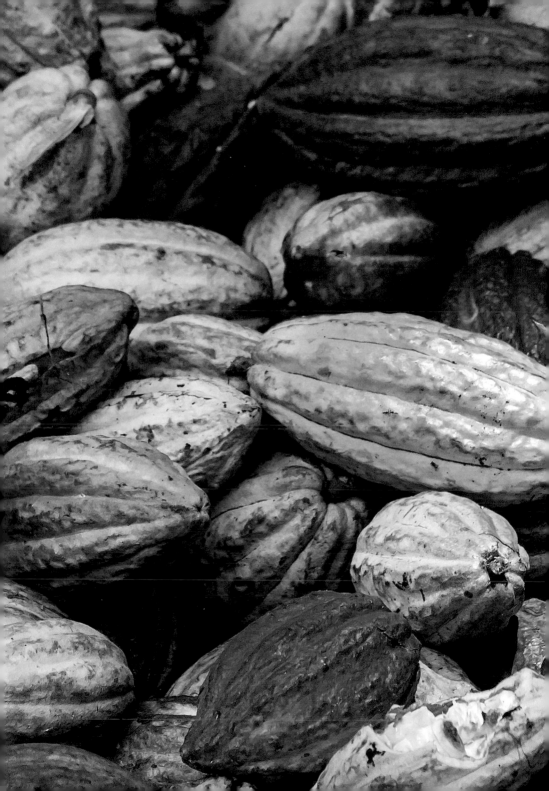

CACAO TRADITIONS: FOOD OF THE GODS

Cacao was part of the Mayan creation myth, Popol Vuh. It was one of the ingredients, along with corn, used by the gods to make the first humans, made by the gods so that they would be worshipped by them. To the Mayans, therefore, cacao was in the essence of humanity, so it became a ceremonial elixir. Due to its aphrodisiac qualities (it contains tryptophan, a building block of serotonin, and phenylethylamine, a part of amphetamine, which are both associated with good mood and feelings of falling in love), Maya couples would drink cacao at engagement and marriage ceremonies.

Archaeological vessels found in tombs from the Mesoamerican period also found cacao cooked with turkey and fish, suggesting that cacao was originally considered to be a savory instead of a sweet ingredient, which makes sense when you taste raw cacao. It was the Spanish who began to serve cacao as a hot and sweet beverage, and in the 1700s, when hot cacao hit London, cacao houses sprang up just as artisan coffee shops are in abundance today.

Aztec mythology

In Aztec mythology, the god named Quetzalcoatl brought down the cacao tree from heaven to earth. This is why the beverage made from dried and fermented cacao beans was thought to bring wisdom.

The Aztecs drank cacao cold, made with corn, chili, and vanilla. Achiote, another spice, was used to give the cacao drink a red color.

Opposite: A depiction of the Aztec god Xiuhtecuhtli from the Codex Fejérváry-Mayer, 15th century.

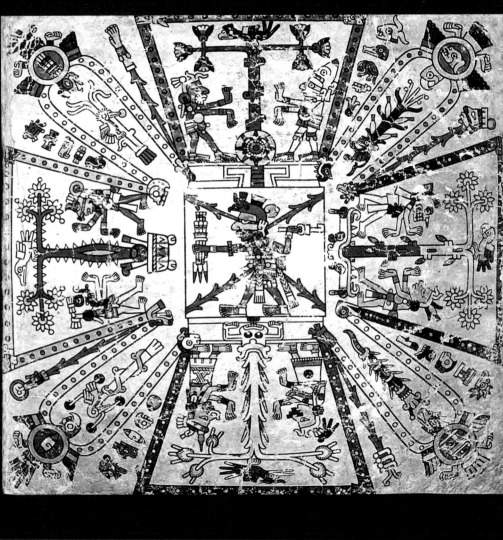

THE CACAO CEREMONY

According to Rebekah Shaman, who gives shamanic guidance and offers ceremonial events, including cacao ceremonies, cacao is also a powerful plant medicine that has been used in ceremonies for millennia across Central and South America, especially by the Mayan people, who believed that cacao was discovered by the gods. The word "cacao" itself originates from the Maya words *kak'au* and *chokola'j*, which combine to mean "to drink chocolate together."

"Cacao has many amazing, life-affirming qualities that support health and psychological well-being. She is a powerful Plant Medicine that helps us to release emotional blockages that no longer serve us, find forgiveness in ourselves and others, and shows us the way forward if we are stuck, or afraid of making necessary life changes. It also enables us to access stuck emotions, conditionings, patterns of behavior, and addictions that are buried deep in the unconscious."
—Rebekah Shaman

The cacao ceremony, now becoming more popular across the world, is thought to create an euphoric state in which the release of negative energy, connection with heart energy, and personal or spiritual transformation can take place. Ceremonies will vary in their approach, depending on the shaman conducting the ceremony. They usually take place in a circle with prayer, sharing intention, and the cacao is served as a beverage. Ceremonial grade cacao is used and it is often mixed with water, chili, and honey or herbs.

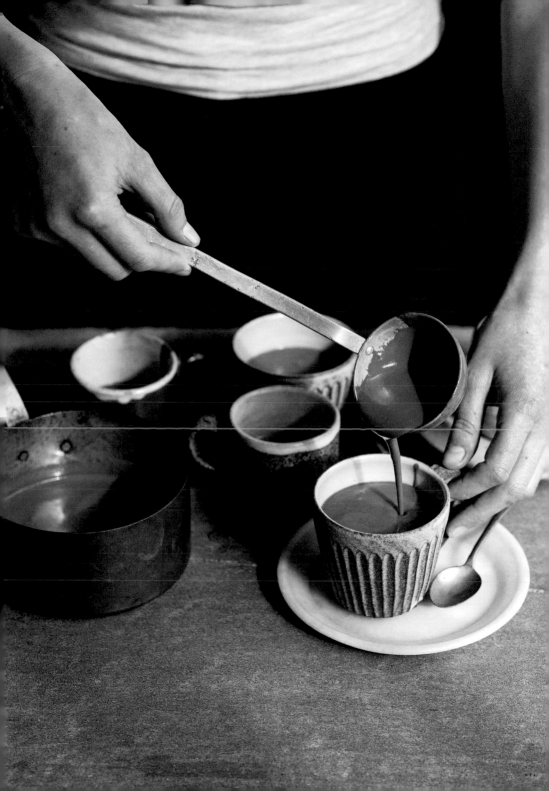

THE HEALTH BENEFITS OF CACAO

It's official. Chocolate is good for us. Or actually, raw, cold-processed cacao is particularly good for us. Cacao powder, or nibs, are healthier than cocoa powder, because all the natural nutrients of the cacao bean are retained, so it has naturally high levels of flavanols, fiber, and protein. Cacao is also said to be one of the highest sources of antioxidants of all foods. Raw cacao contains a number of beneficial minerals and chemicals that are good for our health, from helping to balance blood sugar, to maintaining heart health, brain health, and healthy weight loss.

ANTIOXIDANTS
Raw cacao contains more than 40 times the antioxidants found in blueberries. Antioxidants absorb the free radicals that we are exposed to from pollution and toxins in our environment, causing cell and tissue damage and often leading to diseases, such as cancer.

IRON
Cacao is the highest plant-base source of iron with 7.3mg per 100g (in comparison spinach, which has 3.6mg per 100g). As is the case with all plant-base iron, it is best combined with vitamin C to aid absorption into the body.

MAGNESIUM
Cacao is also a plant-base source of magnesium, which is needed for optimum muscle and nerve function.

CALCIUM
Although you probably won't consume 100g raw cacao instead of drinking ½ cup of cow milk, it is worth noting that cacao contains 160mg calcium per 100g compared to 125mg per 100ml (about ⅜ cup) milk.

MOOD BOOSTER

Cacao is a source of both serotonin and tryptophan, two of the key "good mood" chemicals. It also triggers the release of dopamine and endorphins, thanks to phenylethylamine and anandamide, also known as the "bliss molecule." These chemicals help to relieve emotional stress and produce a natural sense of pleasure.

FIBER AND MUFA

Cacao is a good source of fiber and monounsaturated fats or MUFAs, the healthy fats that keep you fuller for longer and help to lower cholesterol and reduce the risk of heart disease and stroke.

IF YOU ARE SENSITIVE TO CAFFEINE

Cacao beans contain theobromine, which is a nervous system stimulant that has a similar effect to caffeine; it's the ingredient that makes chocolate unsafe for dogs. If you are sensitive to caffeine, you should be careful of how much, if any, cacao you consume.

Next page: Cacao pods on a tree, Brazil

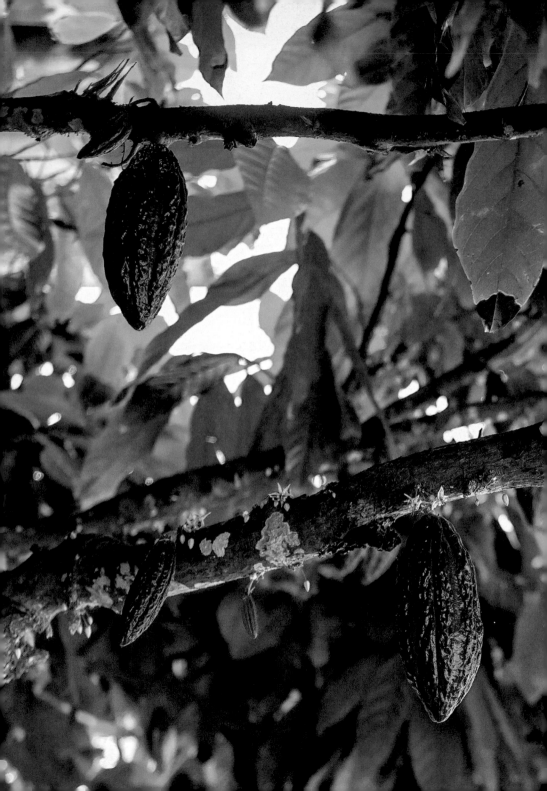

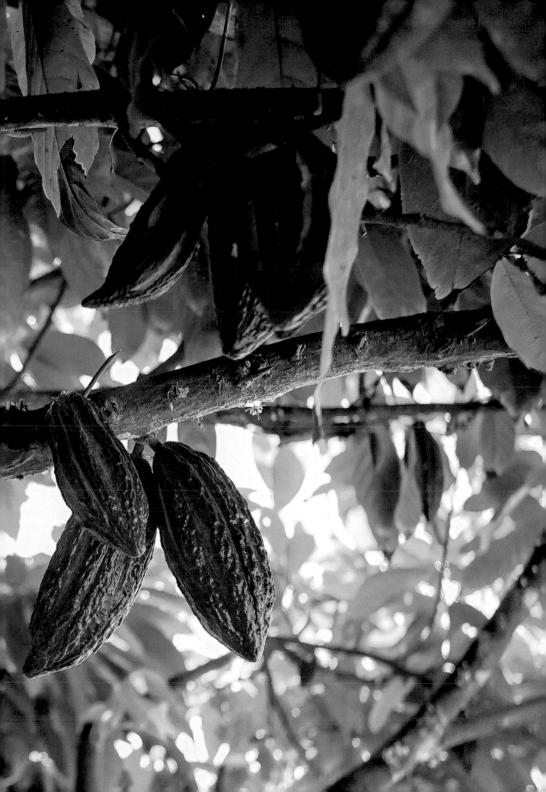

COOKING WITH CACAO

We tend to think of desserts and baking when we first think of cacao or cocoa, and especially when we think of chocolate. However, because raw cacao is unsweetened, it works well in savory dishes as well as sweet, and chefs and flavor experts suggest that it works particularly well with spices, especially chili, cardamom, wasabi, clove, and cinnamon. It can be paired with meats, including beef, pork, steak, venison, and duck, as well as shellfish, beets, and certain cheeses, including ricotta and Parmesan. That is why you will find some slightly unusual sounding combinations in this collection of cacao recipes.

Here are some of the ways in which you can use the different types of cacao in your cooking:

- Add a few shavings of solid cacao to stews to add a wonderful extra layer of flavor.
- Use the nibs as a healthy alternative to chocolate chips, perfect for your morning oatmeal. They are often toasted to boost the flavor (see opposite).
- Add a spoonful of cacao powder to your favorite smoothie for an extra hit of antioxidants.
- Make your own chocolate with cacao butter.
- Break off a square of solid cacao chocolate to make a healthy hot chocolate beverage.

The majority of the recipes in this book avoid cooking cacao at high temperatures, because heat affects the nutrient content, although we couldn't resist a traditional brownie recipe, with a few chia seeds thrown into the mix. There are also a few variations of some traditional cacao recipes from around the world, including the Mexican mole and hot cacao, picada sauce from Spain, and "chocolate salami" from Portugal.

TOASTED CACAO NIBS

If you haven't tasted a raw cacao nib and you imagine they taste anything like what we know of as "chocolate," think again! Because they contain no sugar, nibs are bitter. One easy way to boost the flavor of cacao nibs is to toast them.

- Preheat the oven to 350°F.

- Spread the cacao nibs out on a baking sheet and bake for 10 minutes.

- Remove from the oven and cool completely before using.

- Store in an airtight container.

BEVERAGES

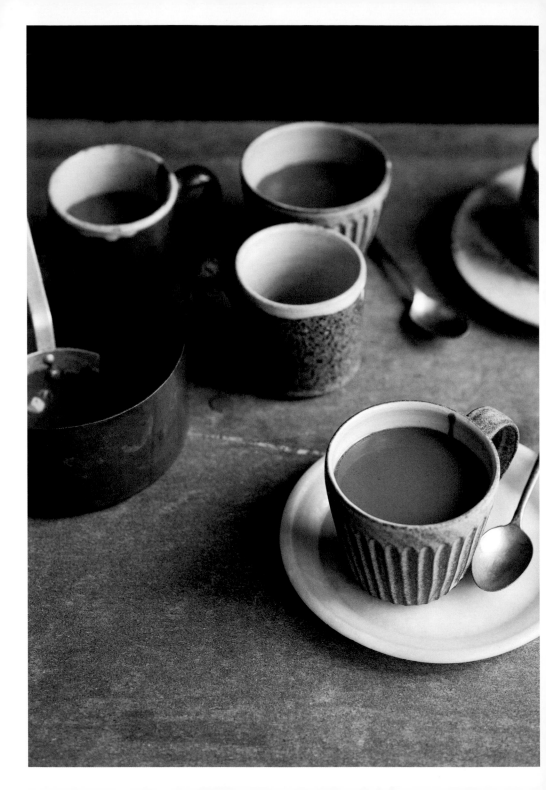

HOT CACAO

In South America, you'll find an amazing variety of hot chocolate recipes, among them *tascalate* (or *tazcalate*), which is made with ground roasted corn, chocolate, ground pine nuts, achiote, vanilla, and sugar. All the ingredients are ground together, mixed with milk, and heated; for a cold drink, the ingredients are stirred into cold water and added to ice. Another tradition is to add chili to hot chocolate. Here, we have combined the antioxidants of cacao with turmeric, famed for its anti-inflammatory properties. The coconut oil helps to emulsify the raw cacao so that you get a silky consistency.

1²/₃ cups almond milk
1 tablespoon coconut oil
1 tablespoon cacao powder
½ teaspoon raw maca powder
½ teaspoon ground turmeric
3 pinches of ground cinnamon
pinch of cayenne
pinch of sea salt

Heat the almond milk and coconut oil in a saucepan. Mix a little of the warm milk with the rest of the ingredients to form a smooth, loose paste. Add it to the rest of the milk and whisk to combine all the ingredients before serving.

TONIC

This is a wonderfully refreshing and light drink. If you can find blood orange juice, the color is intense; however, any citrus juice will work well with this recipe.

---

1 teaspoon cacao powder

1 teaspoon maple syrup

juice of an orange

1 cup blood orange juice
  (or orange juice)

2 cups tonic water

Make a paste with the cacao powder, maple syrup, and juice of an orange. Mix into the the blood orange juice and tonic water and serve over plenty of ice.

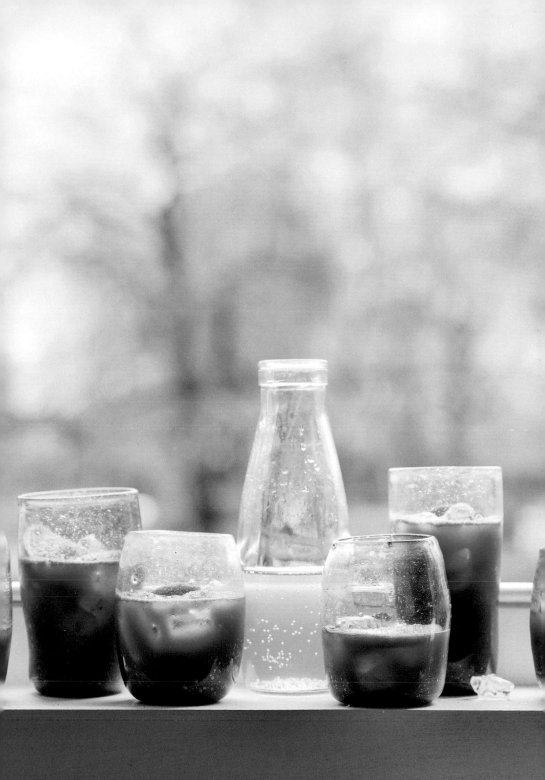

ACAI CACAO SMOOTHIE

Acai smoothies have become a famous export from Brazil—the palm trees from which the berries are harvested are mostly native to Central and South America. Acai and cacao are a classic, luxurious combination.

---

1 tablespoon acai berry powder

1 tablespoon cacao powder

1 frozen banana, sliced

generous handful of frozen
   blueberries

1 tablespoon almond butter
   (optional)

1 tablespoon ground flaxseed

⅔ cup almond milk, plus extra
   if needed

Put all the ingredients into a blender and blend until smooth.

Add a little more almond milk if you like a thinner consistency.

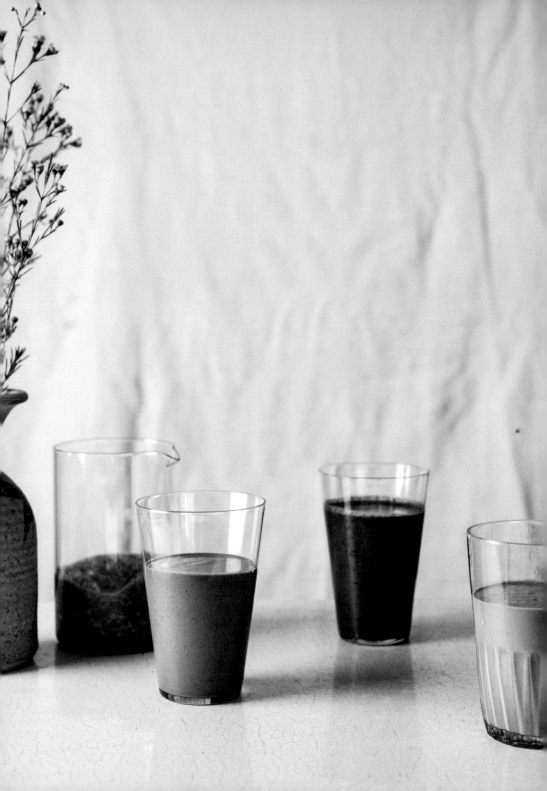

CACAO MATCHA SMOOTHIE

Matcha is another amazing source of antioxidants, and avocado adds healthy monounsaturated fats to this smoothie, so you'll feel fuller for longer. We have also included kefir in this recipe, a type of fermented milk that is packed with beneficial bacteria, but if you don't have it on hand, you can use any type of nut milk or some apple juice instead.

½ frozen banana, sliced

1 tablespoon cacao powder

1 teaspoon matcha powder

handful of spinach

½ ripe avocado, peeled
   and pitted

½ cup kefir

Put all the ingredients into a blender and blend until smooth.

Add a little water if you prefer a thinner consistency.

PEANUT BUTTER CHIA

This high-protein smoothie will power up your morning,
and the peanut butter will really keep you going, especially
after a workout.

---

1 tablespoon peanut butter

2 tablespoons plain yogurt

1 tablespoon soaked chia seeds
   (1 teaspoon dry seeds soaked
   overnight in ¼ cup water)

½ frozen banana, sliced (or use
   3 tablespoons frozen berries)

1 tablespoon cacao powder

⅔ cup coconut milk

Put all the ingredients into a blender and blend
until smooth.

BREAKFASTS

OATMEAL OF THE GODS

The pumpkin in this recipe might not sound like a natural breakfast ingredient, but believe us when we say this is delicious, especially with the flavors of maple syrup, cacao, clove, and cinnamon.

½ cup rolled oats (use gluten-free oats if you are intolerant)

½ cup milk of choice

1 tablespoon pumpkin puree

1 tablespoon maple syrup or honey

¼ teaspoon ground cinnamon

1 teaspoon cacao powder

pinch of ground cloves

1 tablespoon plain yogurt or dairy-free coconut yogurt

a few pieces dried mango

1 tablespoon Cacao Nuts and Seeds (*see* page 57)

Put the oats, milk, and ½ cup water into a saucepan and bring to a boil.

Reduce the heat to a simmer and stir in the pumpkin puree, maple syrup or honey, cinnamon, cacao powder, and cloves.

Simmer gently for about 10 minutes, stirring every now and then, until the oats are soft.

Let stand for a couple of minutes before serving with a spoonful of yogurt, dried mango, and some Cacao Nuts and Seeds.

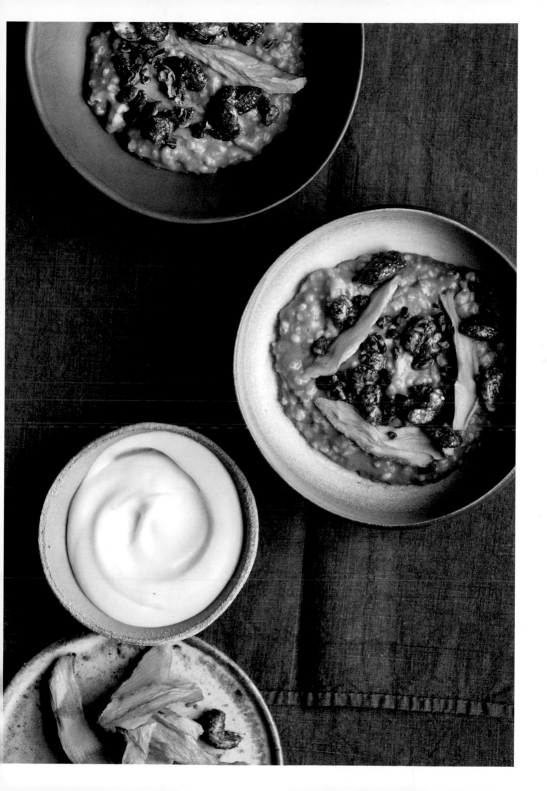

GRANOLA

Whenever we make a batch of granola, we wonder why we don't do it all the time, because it's so easy; it's also difficult to make a bad flavor combination choice when it comes to granola. So if you have almonds instead of hazelnuts, go ahead and use almonds; likewise, if you have a package of dried apricots you want to finish off, you can swap them for the dried berries.

2¾ cups rolled oats

1⅓ cups coarsely chopped
hazelnuts

⅓ cup pumpkin seeds

2 tablespoons cacao powder

2 heaping tablespoons coconut oil
(when solid)

3 tablespoons maple syrup

1 teaspoon vanilla extract

¾ cup dried blueberries or
cranberries

2 tablespoons cacao nibs

Preheat the oven to 275°F and line a large baking sheet with parchment paper.

Mix together the oats, nuts, seeds, and cacao powder in a large bowl.

Heat the coconut oil and maple syrup in a small saucepan until dissolved, and mix in the vanilla extract. Pour the oil and maple syrup mixture into the dry ingredients and stir thoroughly so that all the oats, nuts, and seeds are evenly coated.

Pour the granola onto the parchment paper and spread out evenly. Bake for about 45 minutes, then sprinkle with the dried berries and cacao nibs and bake for another 10–15 minutes.

Let cool and then gently bring up the sides of the paper to transfer the granola to a large airtight jar.

OVERNIGHT OATS

Soaking oats overnight means that you have a quick base for a delicious breakfast the next morning. This recipe is based on a Swiss-style Bircher muesli, which is traditionally served cold, but you could heat up the oats for a warming oatmeal.

½ cup rolled oats (use gluten-free oats if you are intolerant)

1 teaspoon flaxseed

1 teaspoon chia seeds

1 tablespoon cacao powder

²/₃ cup almond milk (or milk of choice)

1 tablespoon maple syrup (optional)

3 drops of vanilla extract

To serve

juice of ½ lime

2 tablespoons plain yogurt (or dairy-free coconut yogurt)

½ apple, chopped

1 tablespoon coarsely chopped almonds

1 teaspoon toasted cacao nibs (see page 19)

Combine all the dry ingredients in a large bowl, add the almond milk, maple syrup (if using), and vanilla extract, and stir thoroughly. Transfer to an airtight glass container and let soften overnight.

To serve, stir through the lime juice, yogurt, chopped apple, and almonds. Finish by sprinkling with the toasted cacao nibs.

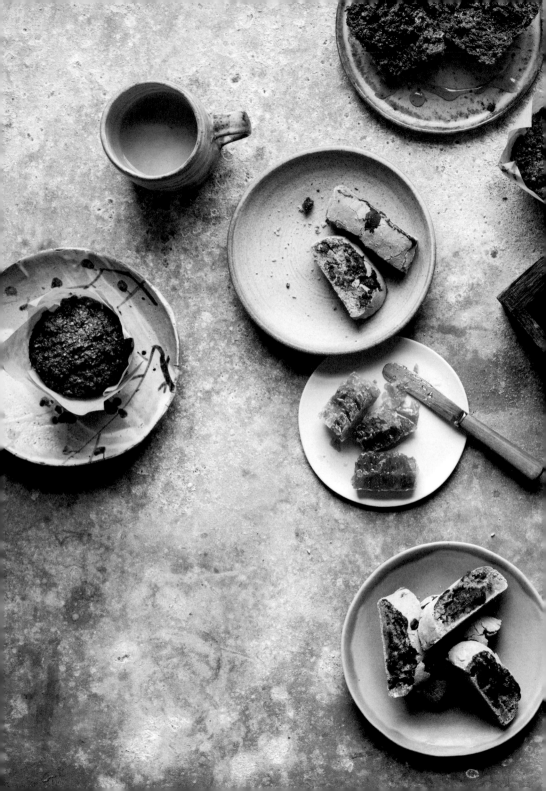

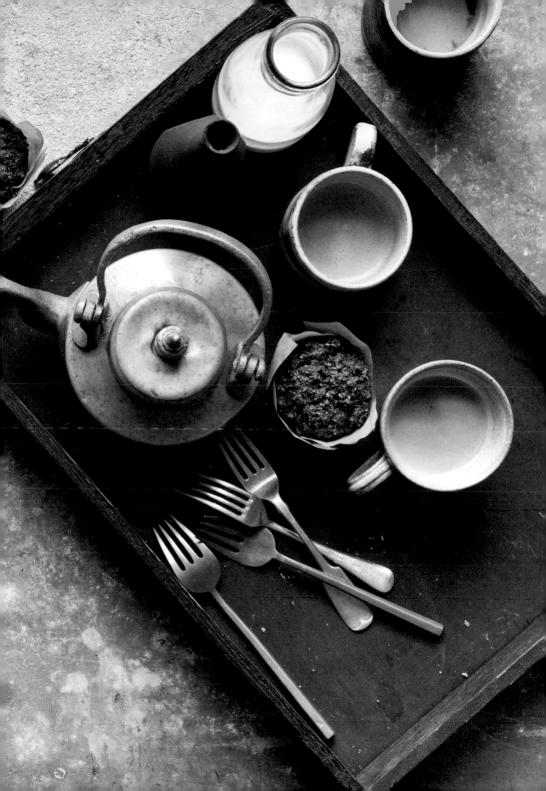

BRAN MUFFINS

The blackstrap molasses and cacao powder make these muffins not for the faint-hearted; they are dark, bittersweet, and delicious warm with a little extra butter.

1¾ cups wheat bran

1 cup raisins

1 cup spelt flour

1 tablespoon cacao powder

1 teaspoon baking powder

1 teaspoon baking soda

1 teaspoon sea salt

5 tablespoons butter

3½ tablespoons coconut palm
   sugar or dark brown sugar

2 tablespoons blackstrap molasses

2 tablespoons honey

1 teaspoon vanilla extract

2 eggs

1 cup Greek-style yogurt

Preheat the oven to 350°F and line a large baking sheet (or two) with parchment paper. Line large 6-cup muffin pan (or a regular 12-cup muffin pan) with paper liners.

Spread out the wheat bran evenly across the lined baking sheet and toast in the oven for 10 minutes, checking to make sure it doesn't burn. Set aside to cool.

Put the raisins and ¾ cup water into a saucepan and simmer over low heat until all the water has been absorbed by the raisins. Remove the raisins from the pan and set aside to cool.

Sift the flour into a bowl and mix through the cacao powder, baking powder, baking soda, and salt. In a separate bowl, use a handheld electric mixer to cream together the butter and sugar until fluffy. Add the molasses, honey, and vanilla and mix again until just combined. Add the egg and mix briefly until just incorporated. Add the yogurt and drained raisins and mix until just combined.

Add the dry ingredients to the wet and mix together until thoroughly combined to make a batter. Pour the batter into the paper liners and bake in the oven for 20–25 minutes or until a toothpick pierced in the center of the muffins comes out clean. Larger muffins will take a little longer. Transfer the muffins to a wire rack to cool completely.

◇◇◇◇◇◇

GINGER AND CACAO BISCOTTI

Perfect for dipping in a cup of hot cacao or coffee, the best thing about making your own biscotti is that you can decide what size you want to make them. Also, we like to bake them just a little softer than regular biscotti.

1 extra-large egg

¼ cup coconut palm sugar or dark brown sugar

1 cup all-purpose flour, plus extra for dusting

½ teaspoon baking powder

1 teaspoon ground ginger

½ teaspoon ground turmeric

⅓ cup cacao drops

Preheat the oven to 340°F and lightly grease a baking sheet.

Beat the egg and sugar with a handheld electric mixer for about 5 minutes, until frothy and leaving a ribbon trail in the mixture.

Add the dry ingredients and combine thoroughly to form a sticky ball of dough. Lightly dust your hands with flour and work the dough into a log about 12 inches long. Place the log on the baking sheet, flatten slightly, and bake in the oven for 20 minutes.

Remove from the oven and cut the log into ¾-inch slices. Place each biscotti back on the baking sheet and return to the oven for 8–10 minutes or until golden.

Let the biscotti cool completely. You can eat them immediately or store in an airtight container for about a week.

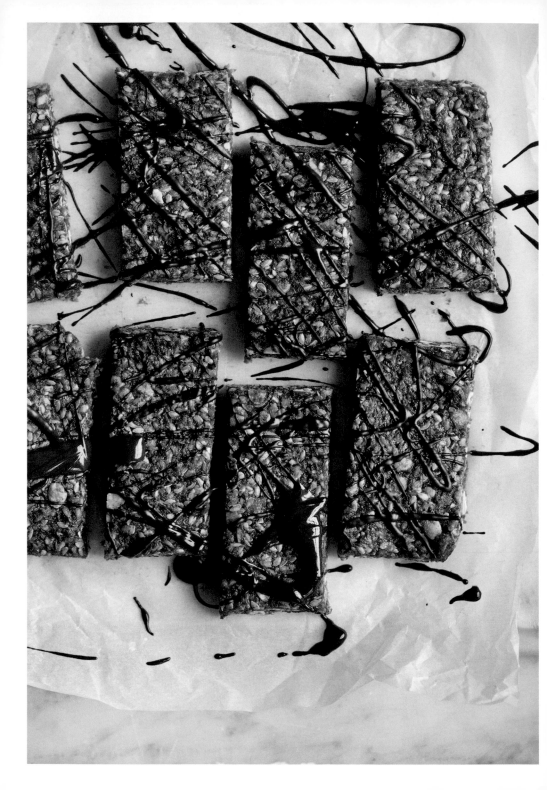

PROTEIN BREAKFAST BARS

These breakfast bars are perfect to make for a busy week ahead, packing in plenty of nutrients. The seeds are the star of the show here, and we've added beet powder, because it goes wonderfully with the cacao, but you could try also try using matcha powder.

¾ cup pumpkin seeds

½ cup flaxseed

7 soft pitted dates

18 soft dried apricot halves

2 tablespoons extra virgin
coconut oil

1 tablespoon cacao powder

1 tablespoon beet powder

pinch of sea salt

1¾ oz cacao, melted (optional)

Line a small baking pan with parchment paper.

Put the pumpkin seeds into a food processor and grind for only a couple of seconds. Pour the chopped seeds into a large mixing bowl and combine with the flaxseed.

Put the dates, apricots, and coconut oil into the food processor and process until you have a paste. Combine the date paste with the seeds. Add the cacao powder, beet powder, if using, and sea salt and stir until the mixture sticks together.

Press the dough into a the prepared pan, then put into the freezer for at least 2–3 hours. Remove from the pan and peel off the paper. Cut into small bars and drizzle with the melted cacao, if using.

The bars will keep in the refrigerator in an airtight container for up to a month, ready to eat whenever you need one.

CACAO BRAZIL NUT BUTTER

This recipe would work equally well with hazelnuts, peanuts, almonds, or cashew nuts. Or for a really simple option, simply stir some cacao powder and coconut syrup or agave nectar through your nut butter of choice.

2¾ cups Brazil nuts

2 tablespoons cacao powder

3 tablespoons avocado oil

⅓ cup coconut syrup or agave
    nectar

pinch of sea salt

1 tablespoon chopped pistachios

1 tablespoon pine nuts

Blend together all the ingredients, except for the chopped pistachios and pine nuts, in a food processor or high-speed blender in bursts of about 30 seconds. Keep going for 8–10 minutes, until the oil releases and a smooth paste forms. You will need to scrape down the sides of the bowl or blender a few times.

Stir through the pistachios and pine nuts.

Transfer to an airtight container and keep in the refrigerator for up to a month.

Serve on toast with a little honey drizzled on top.

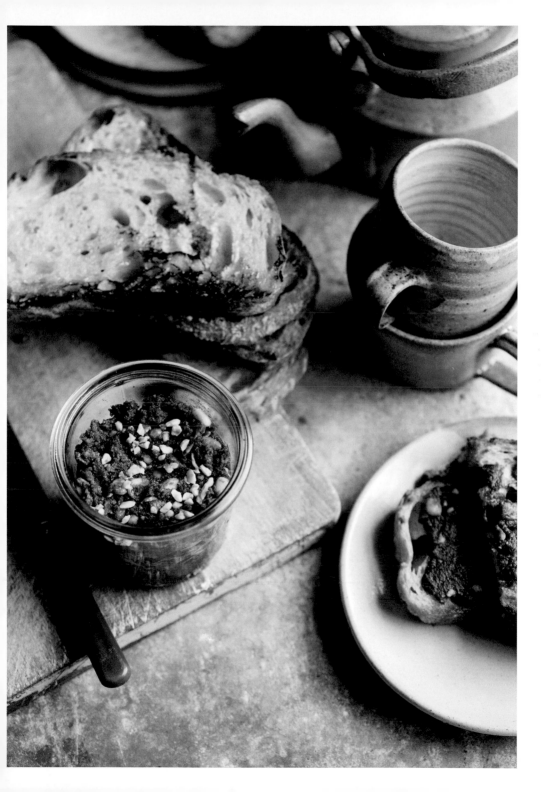

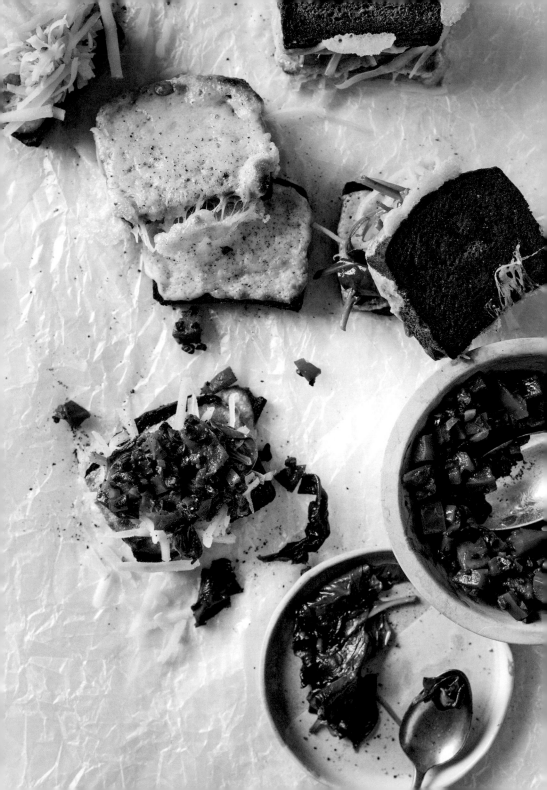

MELTED CHEESE SANDWICH AND CACAO RELISH

According to flavor experts, chocolate and cheese make an unusual but excellent flavor pairing. We've added cacao to a tomato relish for a sweet and savory combination that perks up any melted cheese on toast.

4 slices of rye bread

4 teaspoons unsalted butter

1 cup shredded Comté or Gruyère cheese

3 cups baby spinach

sea salt

For the relish

2 teaspoons butter

1 small onion, diced

2 tomatoes, diced

4 teaspoons cacao nibs

½ teaspoon dried chili flakes

pinch of sea salt

1 tablespoon coconut palm sugar or dark brown suar

To make the relish, put a nonstick saucepan over low-medium heat and add the butter. When bubbling, add the onion, tomatoes, cacao nibs, chili flakes, and salt and sauté for 10 minutes, until soft. Stir through the sugar and continue to heat the relish for another 10 minutes or until it becomes sticky. Remove from the heat and let cool while you make the melted cheese on toast.

Preheat the broiler while you butter the slices of bread on both sides. Toast the bread under the broiler until toasted on each side or use a toaster.

Pile shredded cheese on top of each slice of toast, reserving a little to serve, and place under the broiler until melted and bubbling.

Melt the remaining butter in a saucepan and wilt the baby spinach with a pinch of sea salt.

To make your sandwich, put half the remaining shredded cheese onto one of the cheese toasts. Add a spoonful of relish and some spinach and top with another cheese toast. Repeat to make a second sandwich and devour with a friend.

TURKISH EGGS

We tried adding a little cacao to the traditional Turkish recipe for poached eggs and yogurt—the bitter chocolate works wonderfully with the chili oil. This recipe is perfect when you want something a little more special for the weekend.

splash of white wine vinegar,
    for poaching
4 eggs
¾ cup plain yogurt
1 tablespoon chili oil
½ teaspoon dried chili flakes
1 tablepoon cacao nibs
½ teaspoon sea salt flakes
4 slices of toasted sourdough
    bread, to serve
young peppery greens, to serve
    (optional)

Bring a large saucepan of water to a boil and add a small splash of white wine vinegar. Crack each egg into individual ramekins or small bowls. Stir the water vigorously in one direction and then gently tip the eggs, one by one, into the middle of the water. Poach for 3 minutes, then remove with a slotted spoon and drain on paper towels.

Divide the yogurt between serving bowls. Top the yogurt with the poached eggs and a drizzle of chili oil. Garnish with dried chili flakes and cacao nibs and sprinkle with a little sea salt.

Serve with toasted sourdough bread to dip into the eggs and yogurt, and some young peppery greens, if using.

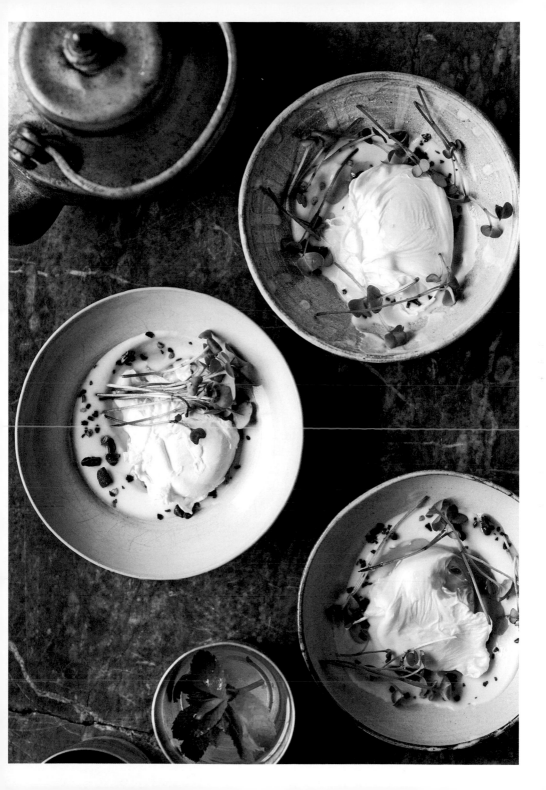

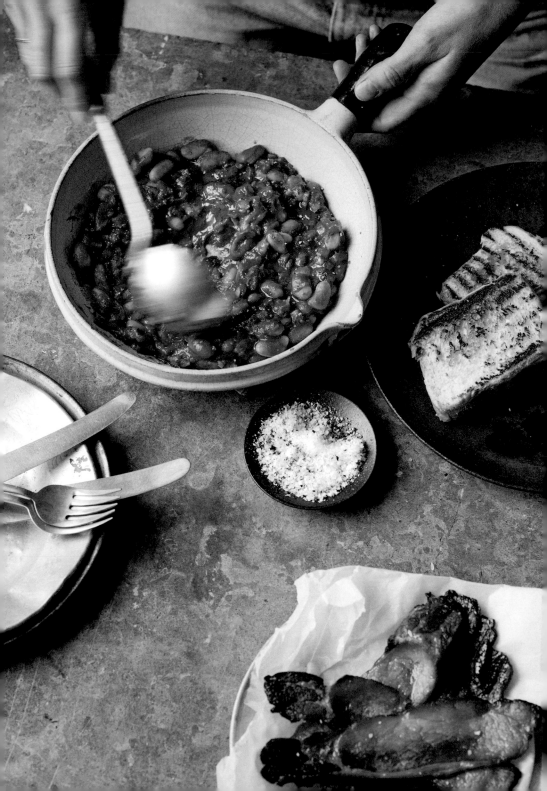

HOMEMADE BAKED BEANS

These beans are delicious and make a protein-packed fulfilling breakfast, lunch, or light dinner. You can top with an egg for Sunday brunch.

2 tablespoons olive oil

½ cup finely diced onion

½ cup finely diced carrots

½ celery stick, finely diced

1 tablespoon tomato paste

1 bay leaf

3 sprigs of thyme, leaves picked

1¼ cups tomato puree or sauce

¼ teaspoon dry mustard

¼ teaspoon ground cloves

2 teaspoons cacao powder

1 tablespoon maple syrup

⅔ cup hot vegetable broth

3 cups rinsed and drained, canned white kidney (cannellini) beans

toasted brioche (or any type of toast) and cooked bacon, to serve

Heat the olive oil in a large lidded casserole or Dutch oven and sauté the onion, carrot, and celery over low-medium heat for about 10 minutes. Stir in the tomato paste, herbs, tomato puree or sauce, spices, cacao, and maple syrup. Add the broth, bring to a boil, then reduce to a simmer and cook for 20 minutes.

Preheat the oven to 350°F.

Add the beans, stir through, put on the lid, and cook in the oven for 20 minutes to combine all the flavors.

Serve on toast with cooked bacon, if you want.

SOUPS & SIDES

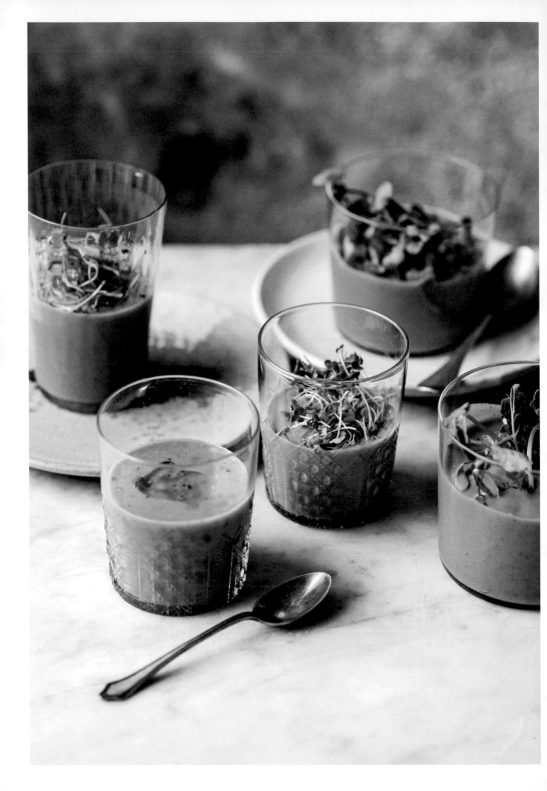

SQUASH, CASHEW NUT, AND CACAO SOUP

The natural sweetness of the butternut squash brings out the flavor of the cacao in this soup. Chili and cacao are natural partners in South America; here, just a hint of a kick brings everything together. We have served it chilled, but it is equally delicious when warmed.

---

1 tablespoon peanut oil

1 small onion, peeled and sliced

½ butternut squash, peeled and coarsely chopped

1 carrot, sliced

2 teaspoons cacao nibs

1 teaspoon mild chili powder

½ teaspoon sea salt

2 cups hot vegetable broth

1 tablespoon cashew nut butter

mixed young peppery greens, to serve

Heat the oil in a heavy saucepan, add the onion, and sauté for about 10 minutes, until translucent. Add the squash and carrot, then stir in the cacao nibs, chili powder, and salt and continue to sauté for another few minutes to let the flavors meld.

Add the hot broth and bring to a boil, then reduce to a simmer and cook for 15 minutes or until all the vegetables are tender. Stir through the cashew nut butter, let cool a little, then blend in a blender until smooth.

Chill in the refrigerator for about an hour.

Serve chilled, sprinkled with young peppery greens.

CAULIFLOWER SOUP
WITH CACAO BUCKWHEAT

The traditional cauliflower soup base in this recipe is light and smooth, so the textures and flavors of the roasted cauliflower, cacao, and roasted buckwheat garnish add a wonderful edge, both visually and in terms of taste. This is so good!

¼ cup olive oil

3 banana shallots, sliced

2 garlic cloves, thinly sliced

2 bay leaves

2 teaspoons thyme leaves

½ teaspoon sea salt

½ cup dry white wine

1 medium-large cauliflower

2 cups hot vegetable broth

2 teaspoons rosemary leaves

1 tablespoon cacao nibs

1 tablespoon honey or maple syrup

2 tablespoons roasted buckwheat

Heat 2 tablespoons of the olive oil in a heavy saucepan and add the shallots and garlic. Soften gently over low heat for 5 minutes, then add the bay leaves, thyme, and salt. After another few minutes, increase the heat and add the wine to the pan.

Remove the outer leaves from the cauliflower. Reserve about one-quarter of the cauliflower and coarsely chop the rest. After the wine has reduced by half, add the chopped cauliflower to the pan. Stir through and sauté for about 5 minutes, then add the hot broth. Bring to a boil, reduce to a simmer, and cook for about 10 minutes, until the cauliflower is easily pierced with a sharp knife. Remove the bay leaves and let cool a little before blending to a smooth soup.

To make the garnish, break the remaining cauliflower into florets and slice them. Put a nonstick sucepan over medium heat and add the remaining olive oil. When hot, add the sliced cauliflower and sauté for a minute, then add the rosemary and cacao nibs. Continue to sauté for another minute or so until the cauliflower is tender. Add the honey and stir through, then add the buckwheat, stirring to combine.

Ladle the hot soup into bowls and top with the cacao, cauliflower, and buckwheat garnish.

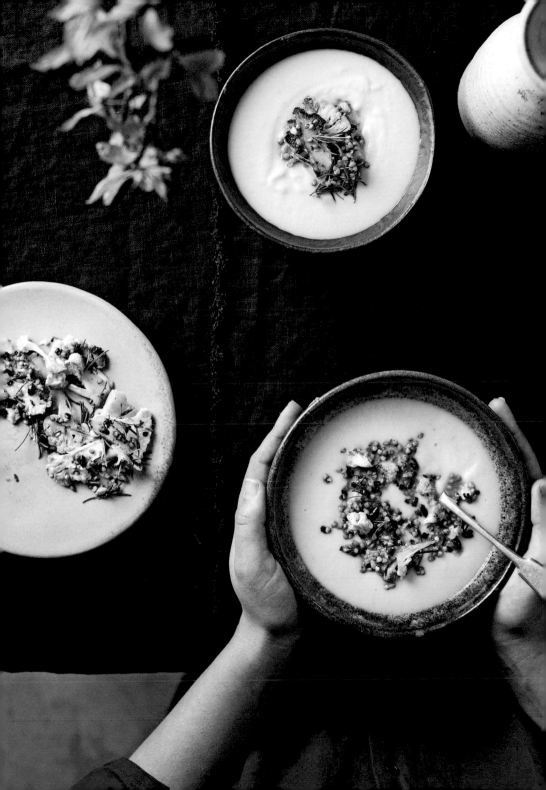

CACAO CHEESE STRAWS
WITH SPICED YOGURT

These cheese straws are hard to resist and are perfect for celebrations
and gatherings. Wasabi is a good flavor companion for cacao, so we
decided to add a little of both here. The spiced yogurt also makes
a great dip for raw vegetables.

For the spiced yogurt

1 green chili, seeded and minced

1 teaspoon finely chopped mint
   leaves, plus extra to serve

1 teaspoon snipped chives, plus
   extra to serve

1 garlic clove, finely grated

½ teaspoon ground cumin

½ teaspoon ground cardamom

½ teaspoon ground coriander

1 cup Greek-style yogurt

1 teaspoon cacao nibs

1 teaspoon toasted buckwheat

1 teaspoon chopped hazelnuts

extra virgin olive oil

For the cheese straws

1½ quantities ready-to-bake rolled
   pie dough (made for 9-inch pies)

½ cup shredded cheddar cheese

pinch of wasabi powder or
   dry mustard

1 teaspoon cacao powder

1 egg, beaten

For the spiced yogurt, mix together the chili, herbs,
garlic, spices, and yogurt and let sit for at least 1 hour
(20 minutes at room temperature, then 40 minutes in
the refrigerator) to bring all of the flavors together.

Preheat the oven to 400°F and line a baking sheet with
parchment paper.

Unroll the dough and cover half of each with the
shredded cheddar, wasabi or dry mustard, and cacao
powder. Fold the dough over like a book and roll lightly
with a rolling pin to seal. Cut the dough into ¾-inch
strips, then halve each strip and twist 2 or 3 times. Place
each pastry straw on the lined baking sheet.

Brush the pastry straws with beaten egg and bake in
the oven for 25–30 minutes, or until golden and crisp.
Place the chilled yogurt in a bowl and top with some
herbs, cacao nibs, toasted buckwheat, hazelnuts, and a
drizzle of olive oil. Serve alongside the cheese straws
for dipping.

CACAO NUTS AND SEEDS

Nuts and seeds are packed with goodness, and this simple recipe adds
a wonderful bittersweet crunch against the nuttiness.

¾ cup raw almonds

¾ cup raw cashew nuts

¾ cup pumpkin seeds

¾ cup unsweetened dried coconut

3 tablespoons cacao powder

1 tablespoon finely chopped
    rosemary

1 teaspoon sea salt

¼ cup olive oil

2 tablespoons maple syrup

4 teaspoons coconut palm sugar or
    dark brown sugar

Preheat the oven to 350°F.

Spread the almonds and cashew nuts out evenly on
a baking sheet and toast for 5 minutes. Remove from
the oven and shake the pan a little to help the almonds
roast evenly. Add the pumpkin seeds to the pan and
bake for another 5 minutes, shaking lightly to make
sure they are evenly toasted.

Remove from the oven and let cool for a couple of
minutes before transferring to a bowl. Stir in the
coconut, then add the cacao powder, rosemary, and salt
and mix thoroughly.

In a small saucepan, combine the olive oil, maple syrup,
and coconut palm sugar. Heat gently and once melted
together, pour the mixture over the nuts and seeds,
stirring to evenly coat in the liquid.

Spread out the coated nuts and seeds on the baking
sheet and bake for another 10–15 minutes. Let cool
completely on the pan before transferring to an airtight
jar. These will stay crunchy for up to a week.

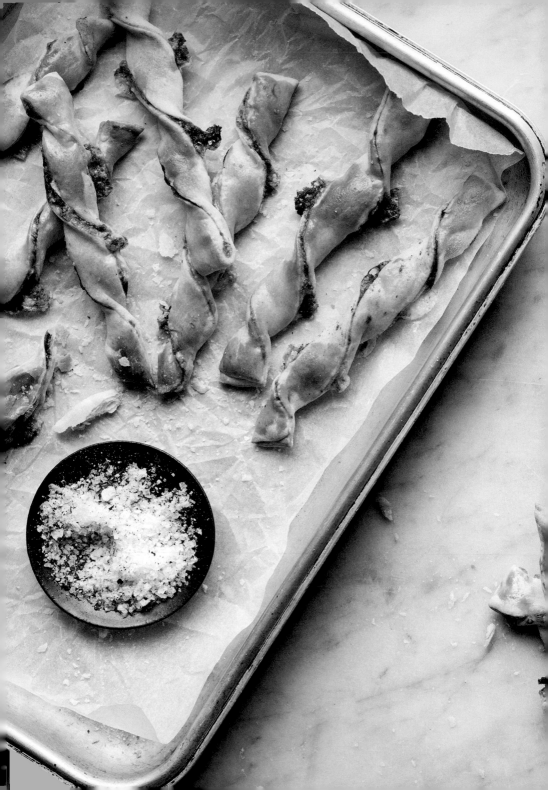

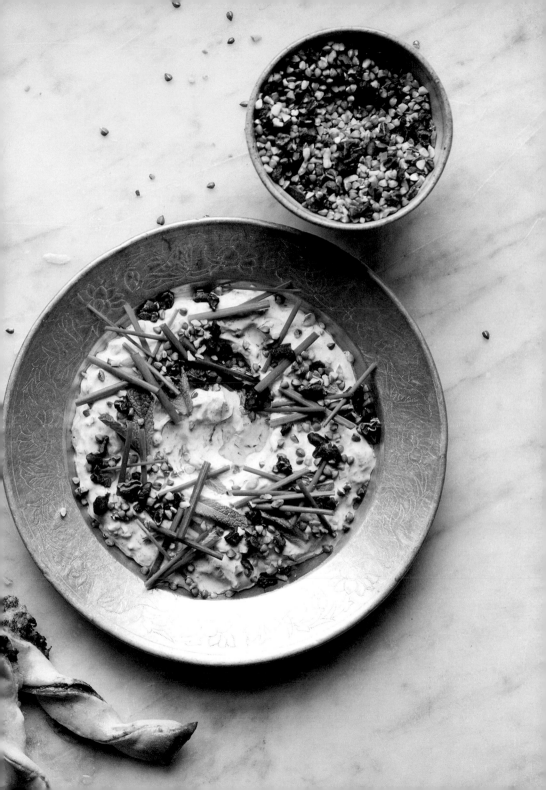

ROASTED CAULIFLOWER
WITH CACAO AND PAPRIKA BUTTER

Roasting cauliflower whole is not only a great way to present this humble vegetable as a sharing dish, but it seems to become sweeter in flavor. We have combined cacao with paprika—which is sweeter and milder than chili—to make a butter to serve with the cauliflower. This dish is delicious served with fish or simply with a grain such as quinoa.

1 cauliflower
2 tablespoons olive oil
3 tablespoons unsalted butter
1 teaspoon sweet smoked paprika
1 teaspoon cacao powder
1 tablespoon cacao nibs
1 tablespoon roasted buckwheat
1 tablespoon chopped hazelnuts
sea salt
handful of leek flowers (optional)

Preheat the oven to 425°F.

Remove some of the outer leaves of the cauliflower and cut the bottom so that it sits flat in a roasting pan. Drizzle with the olive oil and season with salt. Cover it with aluminum foil and roast for about 1 hour in the oven, removing the foil after 30 minutes.

Melt the butter in a small saucepan and add the paprika and cacao powder. Let the spices cook in the butter for a couple of minutes so the flavors can meld.

Serve the cauliflower with the melted butter poured over the top and sprinkle with cacao nibs, roasted buckwheat, and chopped hazelnuts. Season generously and garnish with leek flowers, if using.

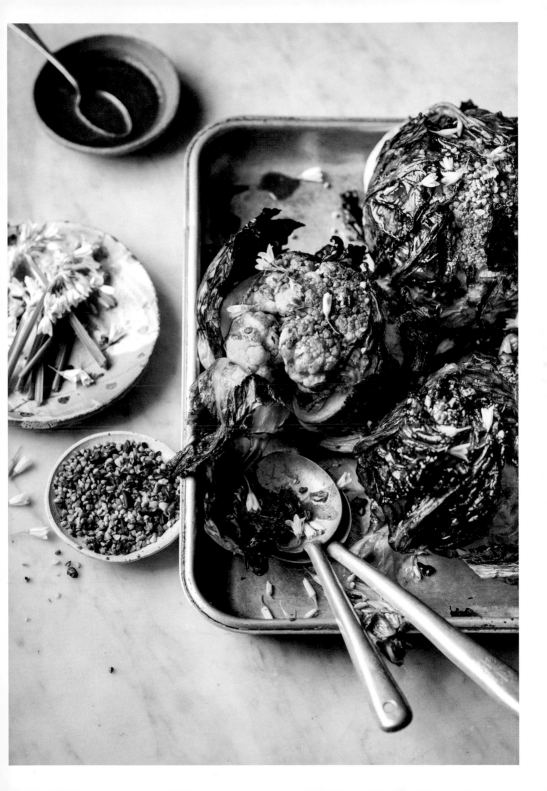

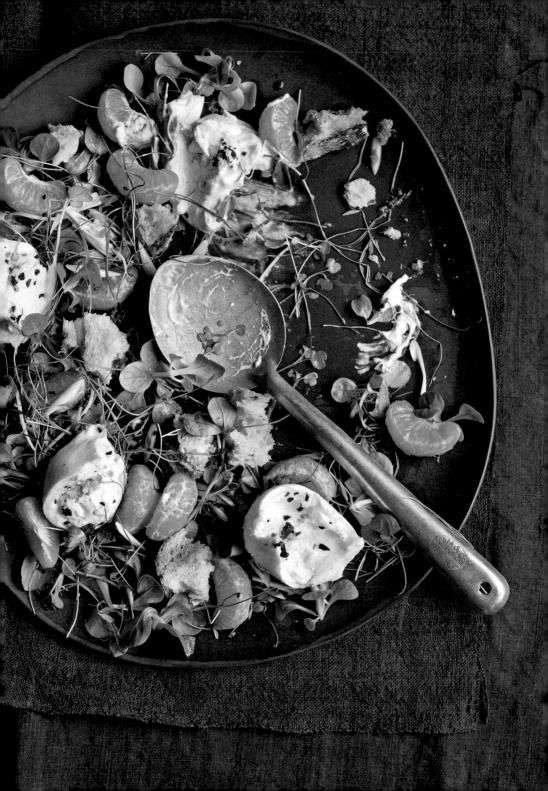

◇◇◇◇◇◇

BURRATA
WITH CLEMENTINE AND CACAO NIBS

This is the simplest of recipes, and it has all the wow factor you need to have friends coming back for more every time.

---

1 tablespoon cacao nibs

½ teaspoon dried chili flakes

1 teaspoon coriander seeds

2 slices sourdough bread, torn into croutons

¼ cup extra virgin olive oil

3 cups corn salad or other greens

¾ cup pea shoots (optional)

2 clementines, peeled and sectioned

2 burratas (Italian balls of mozzarella filled with cream), torn into pieces

sea salt

Put the cacao nibs, chili flakes and coriander seeds into a dry skillet and toast for a minute or two over low-medium heat. Remove from the pan and let cool.

To make the sourdough croutons, preheat the oven to 400°F and line a baking pan with parchment paper. Toss the sourdough pieces in half the olive oil and spread out on the parchment paper. Bake for 10 minutes, until crisp.

Arrange the leaves, clementine sections, and burrata pieces in a large, shallow serving dish.

Generously drizzle with the remaining extra virgin olive oil and sprinkle with toasted coriander seeds, chili flakes and cacao nibs. Add a sprinkling of sea salt and serve with plenty of crispy sourdough croutons.

CARDAMOM ROASTED SWEET POTATO WITH CACAO AND POMEGRANATE MOLASSES

These sweet potatoes are spicy, sweet, and nutty against the cool sour cream and chives. This recipe is such a simple way to add amazing flavors to humble vegetables.

---

2 large sweet potatoes, halved

1 teaspoon ground cardamom

pinch of sea salt

2 tablespoons olive oil

1 tablespoon pomegranate molasses

1 tablespoon cacao nibs

2 tablespoons sour cream

1 tablespoon finely chopped chives

Preheat the oven to 400°F.

Mix all the ingredients, except for the cacao nibs, sour cream, and chives, in a large bowl, making sure the sweet potatoes are evenly coated with the spices, olive oil, and molasses.

Spread out on a baking sheet and bake for about 30 minutes, turning halfway through, until soft on the inside and caramelized on the outside. Add the cacao nibs for the last 5 minutes.

Serve with a generous spoonful of sour cream and a sprinkling of chives.

BABY KALE AND QUINOA SALAD
WITH FETA AND LIME CACAO DRESSING

This is a beautiful fresh salad with protein-packed quinoa, heritage tomatoes, and a zesty dressing. You can use any combination of salad vegetables you want; for example, try adding some chopped avocado or new-season asparagus.

½ cup black quinoa (or use any type of quinoa), rinsed and soaked in water for 30 minutes

2 mixed heritage tomatoes, halved or quartered

3 cups baby kale

⅓ cup crumbled feta

handful of mint leaves, coarsely chopped

¼ cup extra virgin olive oil

juice of ½ lime

½ tablespoon cacao nibs

sea salt

Drain and rinse the quinoa, then add to a saucepan with about 1¼ cups cold water. Bring to a boil, then reduce the heat and simmer for 12–15 minutes, or until the water has evaporated. Drain thoroughly.

Gently mix the cooked quinoa with the tomatoes, baby kale, crumbled feta, and half the chopped mint.

Make a dressing by whisking together the olive oil, lime juice, cacao nibs, and a good pinch of sea salt. Add it to the bowl, gently tossing the salad to distribute the dressing evenly. Taste and adjust the seasoning with more salt or lime juice.

Divide between two shallow bowls and sprinkle with the remaining mint.

MAIN DISHES

BLACK BEAN AND CORN CHILI SHAKSHUKA

This hearty, veggie chili is packed with flavors and will warm up any weekday dinner. Adjust the levels of heat to suit your taste.

2 teaspoons extra virgin olive oil

1 small onion, finely diced

2 garlic cloves, finely grated

1 tablespoon mild chili powder

2 teaspoons ground cumin

¼ teaspoon chipotle chili powder

1 tablespoon cacao nibs

pinch of salt, or to taste

1½ cups drained and rinsed, canned black beans

1 cup drained and rinsed, canned chickpeas

1 (14½-oz) can diced tomatoes

2 teaspoons lime juice

3 eggs

½ tablespoon olive oil

⅓ cup corn kernels, drained or frozen

sea salt and black pepper

2 scallions, finely sliced, to serve

cilantro, to serve

Preheat the oven to 350°F.

Heat the oil in an ovenproof skillet or Dutch oven (in which you will serve the dish) over medium-high heat. Add the onion and and cook for about 5 minutes, stirring often, until the onion is slightly softened.

Add the garlic, spices, cacao nibs, and salt and cook for about 30 seconds, stirring constantly, until fragrant. Add the black beans, chickpeas, tomatoes, 1¼ cups water, and lime juice. Bring to a boil, then cover, reduce the heat to a gentle simmer, and cook for about 20 minutes, checking occasionally if you need to add some water.

Crack the eggs into the pan and transfer to the oven for 15 minutes or until the eggs are cooked but with soft yolks.

Heat a ridged grill pan, add a little olive oil, and grill the corn kernels.

Bring the pan to the table and serve sprinkled with plenty of freshly ground black pepper, a little sea salt, corn kernels, scallion, and plenty of fresh cilantro.

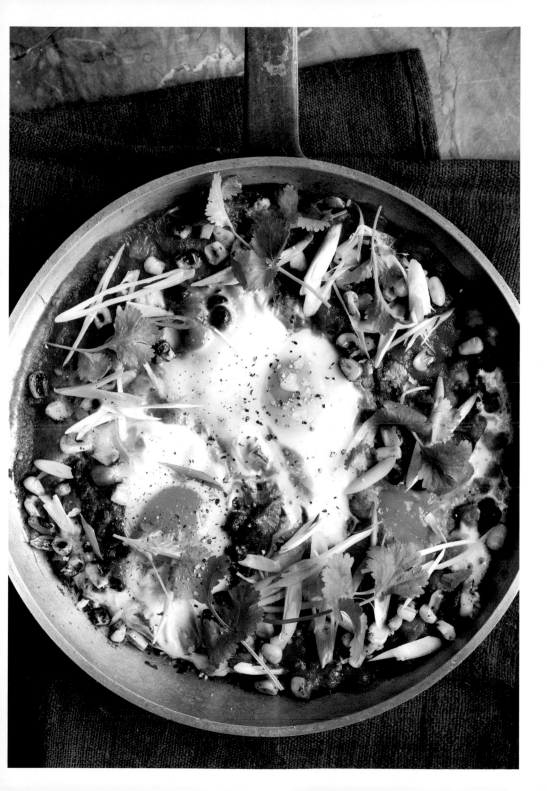

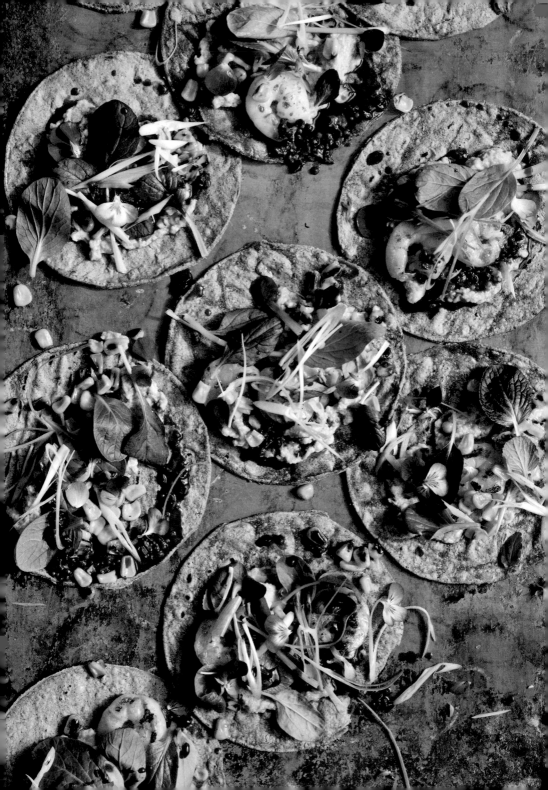

AVOCADO SHRIMP TORTILLAS
WITH BLOOD ORANGE CACAO VINAIGRETTE

This recipe is wonderful for having friends or family around and putting all the elements in the middle of the table so that you can make your own tacos.

---

1 medium avocado

juice of ½ lime (about 1 tablespoon)

½ teaspoon sea salt

½ red chili, seeded and finely
    chopped

1 tablespoon olive oil

7 oz raw and peeled jumbo shrimp

For the dressing

1½ teaspoons cacao nibs

juice of 1 blood orange

1 teaspoon cacao powder

½ teaspoon coconut palm sugar
    or dark brown sugar

2 tablespoons avocado or extra
    virgin olive oil

sea salt

To serve

6 corn tortillas, warmed

1 cup corn kernels, drained

½ cup torn cilantro leaves

2 cups Asian greens or other
    greens of choice

edible flowers, such as violas
    (optional)

lime juice

Halve and pit the avocado and scoop the flesh into a bowl along with the lime juice, salt, and chopped chili. Mash into a guacamole-type texture.

For the dressing, toast the cacao nibs in a dry skillet over medium heat for about 15 seconds. Mix the blood orange juice with the cacao powder and coconut palm sugar, then pour in the avocado or extra virgin olive oil and stir gently to combine. Season to taste with a little sea salt and set aside.

Put a ridged grill pan over medium-high heat and add the olive oil. Season the shrimp with sea salt, and when the pan is hot, grill the shrimp for 20–30 seconds on each side, until just cooked.

To assemble the tortillas, spread some avocado mix over each warm tortilla and top with one or two shrimp. Sprinkle with the corn kernels, cilantro, greens, and edible flowers, if using, and drizzle with the cacao dressing. Squeeze some extra lime juice over the top.

OCTOPUS
WITH MOLE

Mole, from the Aztec word *molli*, meaning "sauce," is the national dish of Mexico. There are many variations, often served with chicken or turkey.

For the mole

2 tomatoes, halved

¼ white onion, halved

½ head of garlic, sliced in half through the middle

2 dried ancho chilies, ribs and seeds removed

2 red chilies, seeded and chopped

⅓ cup sesame seeds

2 tablespoons olive oil

½ teaspoon ground cinnamon

pinch ground cloves

½ teaspoon ground cumin

1 cup chicken broth

2 tablespoons cacao powder

1 tablespoon fine bread crumbs

1 tablespoon maple syrup

sea salt

To make the mole, first preheat the oven to 450°F.

Put the tomatoes, onion, and garlic on a baking sheet and roast in the top half of the oven for 25–30 minutes.

At the same time, soak the ancho chilies in hot water.

When the roasted garlic is cool enough to handle, squeeze the cloves out into a blender, add the other roasted vegetables, softened ancho chilies, and red chilies, and blend until smooth.

Toast the sesame seeds on a baking sheet for a couple of minutes until golden. Let cool, then grind to a powder in a spice mill or mortar and pestle.

Heat the oil in a large saucepan over medium-high heat and cook the ground spices for 30 seconds or until they release their aromas. Add the blended vegetables and chilies, bring to a simmer, and cook for about 5 minutes.

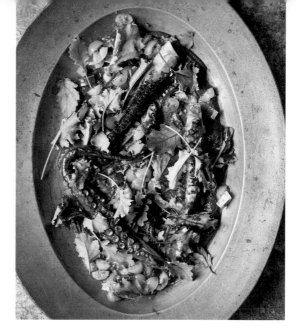

For the octopus

10½ oz octopus tentacles

1 tablespoon olive oil

To serve

baby heritage tomatoes, halved

baby kale

red chili, seeded and finely sliced

extra virgin olive oil

Add the broth, season with a little sea salt, and simmer for about 1 hour, until the sauce is thickened.

Add the cacao, ground sesame seeds, bread crumbs, and maple syrup and whisk gently until incorporated. Cook for another 30 minutes, stirring occasionally. Taste and adjust the seasoning before serving.

To prepare the octopus, bring a saucepan of water to a boil and add the octopus. Simmer for 30 minutes, drain, and rest for another 30 minutes. Toss the octopus tentacles in olive oil, heat a ridged grill pan, and grill the octopus for 3–4 minutes on each side, until charred.

To serve, spread some mole over the bottom of a shallow serving dish. Toss the octopus with the tomatoes, baby kale, and chili along with some extra virgin olive oil and arrange on top of the mole. Season with a little more sea salt and serve.

MACKEREL
WITH CACAO BLACK BEANS

This dish is packed with bold flavors that complement the
mackerel. The puree also goes well with chicken or duck
as a side that adds something a little different.

---

2 mackerel fillets

microgreens, to serve

lime wedges, to serve

For the beans

¾ cup dried black beans, soaked
　in cold water overnight

½ cinnamon stick

1 bay leaf

2 garlic cloves, 1 smashed, 1 sliced

1 tablespoon olive oil

1 small red onion, sliced

¼ teaspoon mild chili powder

1 teaspoon cumin seeds

1 teaspoon coriander seeds

⅓ cup red wine

1 tablespoon cacao powder

1 tablespoon maple syrup

1½ teaspoons apple cider vinegar

1 tablespoon extra virgin olive oil

sea salt

Drain the soaked black beans, rinse in cold water, and
put into a large saucepan with twice their volume of
water. Add the cinnamon, bay leaf, and smashed garlic
clove. Bring to a boil, then reduce to a simmer and cook
for 40–60 minutes, until the beans are cooked and soft,
skimming off any foam that rises to the surface of the
water. Drain, reserving a little of the liquid, and remove
and discard the cinnamon, bay leaf, and garlic clove. Set
the beans aside.

Heat the olive oil in a saucepan over low-medium heat
and add the onion and sliced garlic clove, sautéing for
about 10 minutes. Add the chili powder, cumin, and
coriander seeds and cook for a minute before adding the
wine. When the wine has almost disappeared, add the
cacao powder, maple syrup, and vinegar, then add the
beans to the pan.

Season with sea salt and gently mix all the ingredients
together for a minute or so.

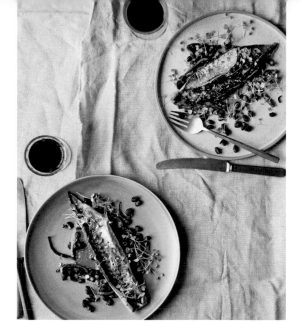

Transfer half the beans to a blender while still warm and add the extra virgin olive oil. Blend, adding a little of the cooking liquid from the beans, if needed, to create a smooth puree. Heat the other half in a nonstick saucepan until the beans begin to pop.

Meanwhile, put a nonstick ridged grill pan over high heat and place the mackerel fillets, skin side down, in the hot pan. Cook for 4–5 minutes, until the skin is crispy, then flip over and after a few seconds remove the pan from the heat. The fillets will finish cooking through in the residual heat.

Divide the bean puree between bowls and top with the rest of the beans and mackerel fillets. Sprinkle with plenty of fresh microgreens and serve with lime wedges for squeezing over the top.

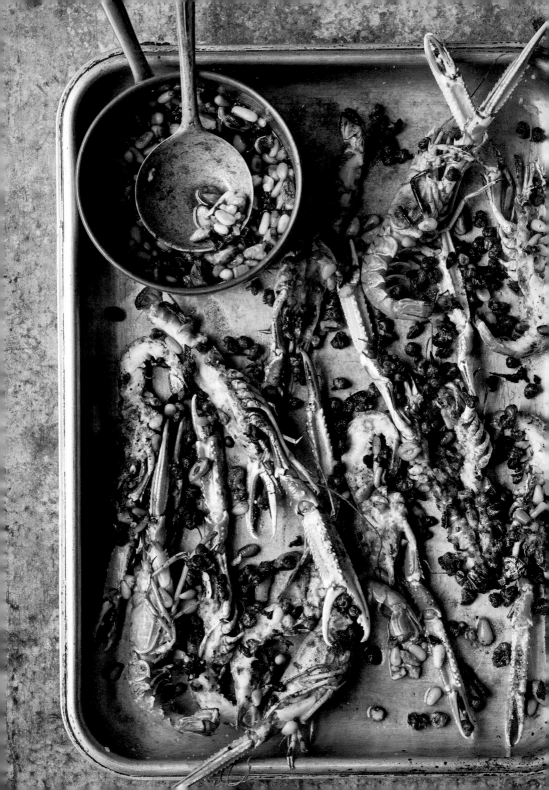

DUBLIN BAY PRAWNS
WITH CACAO BUTTER

This recipe is special. Slicing the prawns through the middle takes a little practice, but as long as you use a sharp knife and make sure you cut away from you, the end result is worth it—buttery broiled prawns that you can simply scoop out of the shells.

⅓ cup olive oil

small pinch of dried crushed chilies

½ garlic clove, finely chopped

1 stick (½ cup) butter, softened

2 tablespoons pine nuts

2 tablespoons hazelnuts, chopped

3 tablespoons cacoa nibs

juice of 1 lemon

16 Dublin Bay prawns (or substitute with larger spiny lobsters or smaller crayfish)

sea salt

Preheat the broiler to its highest setting.

Put the olive oil into a small saucepan, add the dried crushed chilies and garlic, and gently warm over low heat for 2–3 minutes. Remove from the heat, add the butter, and let melt and infuse.

Heat a nonstick skillet, add the pine nuts, chopped hazelnuts, and cacao nibs, and toast for a couple of minutes. Add to the oil and butter infusion along with the lemon juice and whisk to combine.

To prepare the Dublin bay prawns, hold each one firmly down on a cutting board and, using the tip of the knife, score a slit into the head. Then insert the knife completely into the shell and slit the prawn in half lengthwise, making sure you cut away from your body to protect yourself.

Place the prawns, shell side down, on a baking sheet. Pour most of the cool, infused butter over the prawns, season with sea salt, and place under the broiler for 3–5 minutes, depending on size. They will turn from translucent to a pale pinkish white when cooked.

Halfway through cooking, baste them with any remaining butter from the bowl. Serve immediately.

CACAO-CRUSTED COD

The crust in this recipe would also work well with salmon or trout fillets.
It adds a delicious crunch to the dish.

½ cup vegetable broth
16 sprigs of rosemary
1 tablespoon honey
1 tablespoon roasted buckwheat
1½ teaspoons coconut flakes
1½ teaspoons slivered almonds
1½ teaspoons pumpkin seeds
1½ teaspoons mixed sesame seeds
1 tablespoon cacao powder
2 (5½-oz) cod fillets
2 tablespoons olive oil
1 teaspoon Dijon mustard
⅔ cup drained corn kernels
　(defrosted if frozen)
2 tablespoons Greek-style yogurt
sea salt
rosemary flowers, to serve
　(optional)

Preheat the oven to 425°F.

Put the broth into a saucepan with the rosemary and simmer vigorously for about 10 minutes to reduce by about half. Whisk in the honey, then strain to remove the rosemary; keep warm.

Prepare the crust by mixing together the buckwheat, coconut flakes, slivered almonds, pumpkin seeds, mixed seeds, and cacao powder.

Season the cod fillets with sea salt. Heat half the olive oil in a nonstick, ovenproof saucepan over medium-high heat. When hot, add the fillets, skin side down, and sear for 2 minutes. Carefully brush with mustard and top with some of the crust mix before placing the pan in the oven to bake for 5 minutes, or until just cooked (the time will depend on the thickness of the fillets). Rest for a couple of minutes.

Heat the remaining olive oil in a skillet and sauté the corn kernels until slightly charred. Divide between two shallow bowls, top with the cod fillets, and gently pour over some reduced broth. Serve with a spoonful of Greek-style yogurt and a little sea salt to taste.

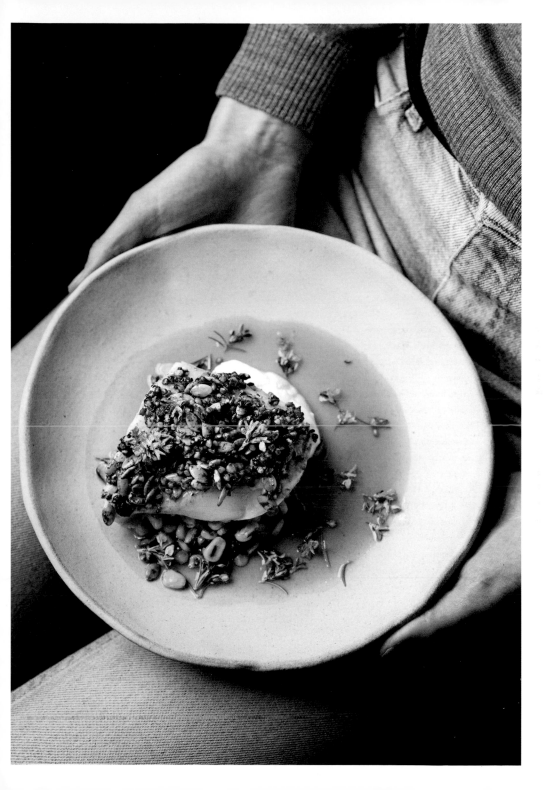

CATALAN CHICKEN PICADA

This is a traditional Spanish dish that combines chocolate with Mediterranean flavors and is usually made with almonds and bread.

---

4 chicken legs

2 tablespoons olive oil

1 onion, finely chopped

2 garlic cloves, finely sliced

1 (14½-oz) can diced tomatoes

1⅔ cups chicken broth

½ cup Spanish sherry

2 bay leaves

3 sprigs of thyme

sea salt and black pepper

For the picada

1 slice of stale sourdough bread, cubed

½ cup slivered almonds

1 oz solid cacao, chopped

pinch of ground cinnamon

pinch of ground cloves

pinch of saffron threads

¼ teaspoon fennel seeds

1 roasted black (or white) garlic clove

¾ cup flat-leaf parsley

extra virgin olive oil

Season the chicken with salt and pepper while you heat the oil in a large saucepan over medium heat. Add the chicken, skin side down, and cook for 3–4 minutes on each side, until the skin is browned. Transfer to a plate and set aside.

Add the onion and garlic to the pan and cook over medium heat for 8–10 minutes, until softened. Add the diced tomatoes and cook for a few minutes until thickened. Add the broth, sherry, bay leaves, and thyme and bring to a boil. Return the chicken to the pan, season with salt and pepper, then cover and simmer over low heat for 30 minutes, turning once during cooking.

Meanwhile, preheat the oven to 350°F. Toast the bread cubes and almonds on a baking sheet for 8 minutes.

Add the toasted bread and almonds to a food processor with the cacao, cinnamon, ground cloves, saffron, fennel seeds, garlic, parsley, and a dash of extra virgin olive oil. Process to a paste, then stir this *picada* into the sauce and simmer over low heat for 15 minutes. Rest for another 10 minutes with the lid on before serving.

PORK BELLY
WITH CACAO GLAZE

This sweet and spicy glaze cuts through the pork and adds a wonderful stickiness.
Don't stand on ceremony with this dish; put it in the middle of the table and be
prepared to move quickly.

2½ tablespoons honey

2 tablespoons olive oil, plus extra
    for grilling

5 garlic cloves, crushed with
    1 teaspoon cacao powder

2 teaspoons sea salt

½ teaspoon ground black pepper

1 dried ancho chili (or 1 red chili,
    seeded)

6½ lb boneless pork belly

2 tablespoons toasted cacao nibs
    (*see page 19*)

Combine the honey, oil, crushed garlic, cacao, salt, pepper, and 3 tablespoons water in a small saucepan and bring to a simmer. Add the ancho chili, if using, and cook for about 8 minutes, until soft. Remove from the heat and let cool before blending in a food processor. If using a fresh chili, cook for only a couple of minutes before blending.

Pour half the glaze over the pork belly and let marinate at room temperature for 1 hour.

Oil a ridged grill pan and put it over high heat. Add the pork and sear over high heat for 2 minutes on each side, then over medium heat for 20–25 minutes, turning it over and glazing every 10 minutes, until the meat can be easily pierced with a knife.

Remove from the heat, place on a board, and let rest for 10 minutes.

Bring the remaining glaze to a boil in a small saucepan, add the toasted cacao nibs, reduce to a low simmer, and cook for a couple of minutes until thickened. Pour the reduced glaze over the pork and carve into slices.

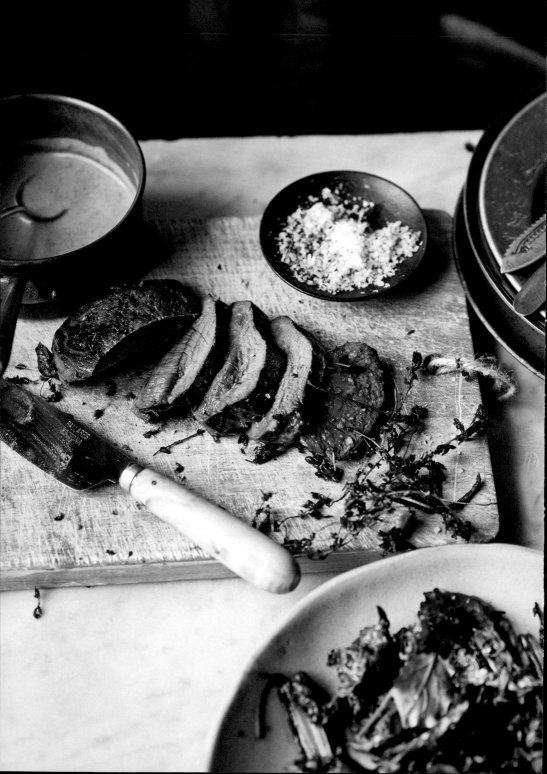

VENISON
WITH CACAO YOGURT

This is Sunday lunch with a difference. Venison is a wonderfully lean and
tasty meat that works really well with the bittersweet yogurt.

For the labneh

⅔ cup natural yogurt

1 tablespoon date syrup

1 tablespoon cacao powder

1 teaspoon sweet smoked paprika

pinch of sea salt

For the venison

1 medium venison tenderloin,
    about 1 lb

1 tablespoon olive oil

3 tablespoons unsalted butter

5 sprigs of thyme

1½ teaspoons cacao nibs

Whisk together the syrup, cacao powder, paprika, and
salt and fold into the yogurt. Let the flavors infuse while
you prepare the venison.

Preheat the oven to 450°F while you bring the venison
to room temperature.

Pat dry the venison with paper towels and season with
sea salt. Heat the oil in an ovenproof ridged grill pan and,
when hot, sear the venison for 2–3 minutes on each side.
Add the butter, thyme, and cacao nibs to the pan and
continue to cook the venison for another 2 minutes,
basting with the melting butter. Give it one final baste,
then place the pan in the oven for 4 minutes.

Remove from the oven and transfer the meat to a board,
carefully pouring any herbed butter in the pan over
the meat. Cover with aluminum foil and let rest for
8 minutes before slicing. Serve with the cacao labneh
and plenty of fresh vegetables.

SERVES 4

◇◇◇◇◇◇

DUCK
WITH CACAO RISOTTO

The cacao in this risotto gives a lovely edge to the sweetness of the
rice, the umami mushrooms, and the richness of the duck.

---

2 duck breasts

2 tablespoons olive oil, plus extra
    for the garnish

1 onion, finely chopped

3 garlic cloves, finely chopped

1⅓ cups risotto rice

3½ oz dried shiitake mushrooms,
    soaked in a small bowl of
    boiling water

4¼ cups hot chicken or vegetable
    broth

1¾ tablespoons butter

1 tablespoon solid (100 percent)
    cacao chocolate shavings

sea salt

1 small onion, sliced

Parmesan shavings, to serve

red microgreens or torn fresh basil,
    to serve

Preheat the oven to 325°F.

Season the duck breasts with sea salt and place them,
skin side down, in an ovenproof skillet. Put the pan
onto the cold stove, then turn on the heat to fairly high.
When the skin is seared and beginning to brown, turn
the breasts over and sear the other side. Turn over again
so the duck is skin side down and place in the oven to
roast for 5–8 minutes, depending on the size of the
breasts. You'll know it's done if it has a just about firm
feel when pressed. Remove from the oven and rest for
a few minutes before slicing. Keep warm.

Meanwhile, start preparing the risotto. Heat the olive
oil in a large saucepan, add the onion and garlic, and
sauté over low heat for about 10 minutes, until soft. Add
the rice and stir to coat in the oil and onion mixture.

Slice the soaked mushrooms and add half, along with
the liquid they were soaked in, to the rice. Bring to
a simmer and stir often until the liquid has been

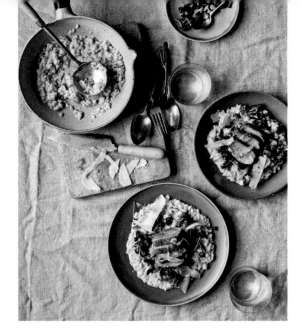

absorbed. Now add a ladleful of broth at a time and
simmer until absorbed; keep going until the rice is
tender. Remove from the heat and stir through the
butter and cacao shavings.

Sauté the onion for 5 minutes in a little olive oil,
add the remaining mushrooms, and sauté for another
5 minutes.

Serve the risotto in shallow bowls topped with the duck
slices and sautéed onions and mushrooms. Season with
a little sea salt and garnish with Parmesan shavings and
microgreens or basil.

BEEF SHORT RIBS
WITH CACAO AND ORANGE

Beef short ribs are inexpensive and delicious when slow cooked
with the bold flavors in this recipe.

---

8 beef short ribs

⅓ cup all-purpose flour

4 bacon slices, cut into ¾-inch
   strips

2 tablespoons olive oil

1 onion, chopped

3 celery sticks, chopped

2 shallots, finely chopped

2 garlic cloves, crushed

½ cup white wine

2 teaspoons soy sauce

2 cups hot chicken broth (enough
   to cover ribs)

zest and juice of 1 orange

2 bay leaves

2 sprigs of thyme

2 teaspoons Chinese five-spice
   powder

1 tablespoon dark brown sugar

1½ tablespoons cacao powder

sea salt and black pepper

Preheat the oven to 350°F.

Season the ribs with salt and pepper, then dredge them
in the flour. Set aside.

In a large casserole or Dutch oven, cook the bacon over
medium heat until crispy and all the fat is rendered out.
Remove the bacon and set aside. Add a glug of olive oil
to the bacon grease left in the pan, then increase the
heat to high. Brown the ribs on all sides before removing
them and setting aside with the bacon.

Reduce the heat to medium, add the onion, celery,
shallots, and garlic, and cook for 2 minutes. Add the wine
and scrape all the sediment from the bottom of the pan
to make sure you keep all those flavors. Bring to a boil
and cook for another couple of minutes.

Add all the remaining ingredients and stir to combine,
then taste to check the seasoning. Return the ribs and
bacon to the pan; they should be completely covered in
liquid, so add more broth, if needed. Cover with the lid

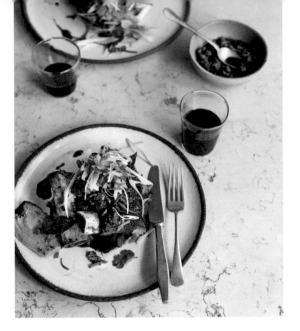

To serve

1 small butternut squash,
    quartered and seeded

2 tablespoons olive oil

1 teaspoon cumin seeds

1 teaspoon caraway seeds

3 scallions, thinly sliced

1 red chili, seeded and thinly sliced

cilantro leaves

and place in the oven for 2 hours, then reduce the heat to 325°F and cook for another 30–45 minutes. The ribs should be fork-tender and beginning to fall off the bone when ready.

Meanwhile, mix the butternut squash quarters with the olive oil, cumin, and caraway seeds. Transfer to a baking sheet and roast in the oven for 30–40 minutes. You can put it in the oven for the last 20 minutes of the beef cooking time and then increase the oven temperature to 425°F, for the remaining 20 minutes, or until the edges are soft and caramelized.

Remove the casserole from the oven and let rest for at least 20 minutes. Skim the fat off the top of the broth before serving.

Serve the beef with the roasted butternut and a sprinkling of sliced scallions, chili, and cilantro.

LAMB RAGU
WITH PAPPARDELLE

This dish is one of our favorites. If you only make one recipe
from the book, let it be this one.

1 tablespoon olive oil

1 onion, chopped

3 garlic cloves, crushed

2 bay leaves

2 tablespoons finely chopped
   oregano

14 oz ground lamb

2 cups lamb broth (or use chicken
   broth)

1 tablespoon tomato paste

1 tablespoon cacao powder

9 oz dry pappardelle

⅓ cup mascarpone

¾ oz solid (100 percent) cacao
   chocolate, finely grated

Parmesan, to serve

wild garlic shoots, to serve
   (optional)

sea salt

Heat the olive oil in a large skillet, add the onion, garlic,
bay leaves, and oregano, and cook, stirring, over medium
heat for about 5 minutes. When the onion is soft, add
the ground lamb and cook until browned all over,
breaking up the lamb with a wooden spoon.

Add the broth and tomato paste, stir through the cacao
powder, bring to a simmer, and cook for 30 minutes,
until the liquid has reduced down.

Cook the pasta in a large saucepan of boiling salted
water according to the package directions. Drain and
refresh under cold running water, then transfer the
pasta to the pan of lamb ragu and toss thoroughly. Finish
with the mascarpone, tossing through before serving.

Serve the pasta in a large serving bowl, with cacao
grated over, Parmesan shavings, and wild garlic shoots.

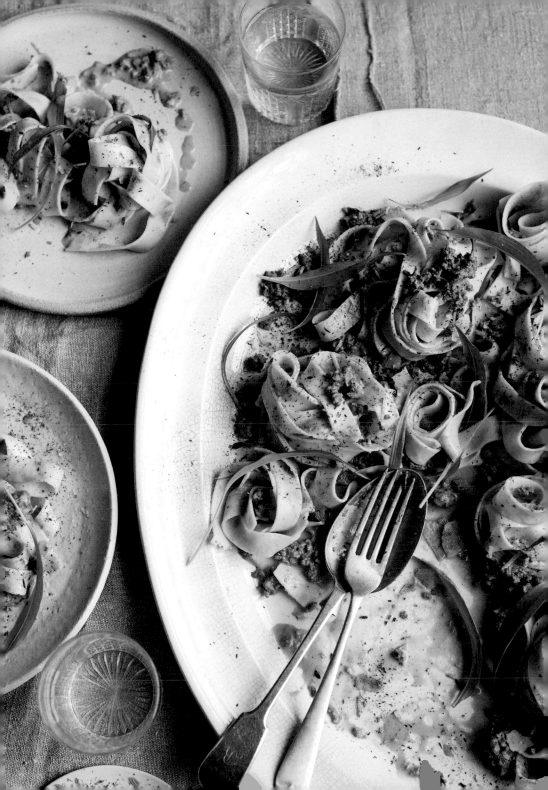

BARBECUE CHICKEN

This sweet, sticky sauce is delicious brushed on chicken, burgers or vegetables on the barbecue.

1 tablespoon olive oil

1 onion, diced

½ teaspoon sea salt

1 tablespoon grated fresh ginger

2 cups tomato puree or sauce

2 tablespoons Worcestershire
    sauce

3 tablespoons honey

3 tablespoons blackstrap molasses

2 tablespoons apple cider vinegar

1 tablespoon cacao powder

1 tablespoon smoked paprika

good pinch of cayenne pepper

4 large or 8 small chicken thighs

For the barbecue sauce, heat the olive oil in a small saucepan over medium heat and add the diced onion and salt. Cook, stirring, for 8–10 minutes, until the onion is caramelized and golden brown, then add the ginger and cook for another few minutes.

Add all the remaining ingredients, except for the chicken, and simmer for about 20 minutes, until the flavors are combined.

Preheat the oven to 375°F.

Marinate the chicken thighs in ¼–⅓ cup barbecue sauce in a bowl for 20–30 minutes. Put into a baking dish and bake in the oven for about 30 minutes. Alternatively, cook on a hot barbecue grill.

Serve with Cardamom Roasted Sweet Potato (*see* page 64, if you want).

ONGLET
WITH MISO CACAO BUTTER

Onglet is a type of steak that is less expensive than rib-eye or tenderloin but with some care and attention is just as tender. The miso cacao butter adds a great umami flavor.

14 oz onglet steak
1 teaspoon white miso
1 teaspoon cacao powder
1 tablespoon olive oil
2 tablespoons unsalted butter
sea salt

Bring the steak to room temperature and season with a little salt. Mix together the miso and cacao.

Put a ridged grill pan over high heat and add the olive oil. When hot, add the steak and sear for 3–4 minutes on each side, turning it often (onglet is more tender when cooked in this way instead of turning it only once after a few minutes).

Remove from the heat and add the butter and miso cacao mixture, spooning it over the onglet as it melts. Let rest for 8 minutes before removing the meat from the pan to slice. Then reheat the butter in the pan and return the steak slices to the pan to just heat through.

Serve with your favorite vegetables or a green salad.

SWEETS

CACAO CHIA PAN BROWNIE

Brownies are one of the easiest cakes to bake—perfect for those times when you just need a chocolaty treat. We've added chia seeds into the mix, although we have to admit the butter and sugar mean this isn't the healthiest recipe; even so, we couldn't resist including them.

---

1 stick (½ cup) butter, plus extra for greasing

1 cup coconut palm sugar or dark brown sugar

1 cup cacao powder

⅓ cup all-purpose flour

½ teaspoon baking powder

¼ teaspoon sea salt

1 teaspoon vanilla extract

2 extra-large eggs

2½ tablespoons chia seeds

1 tablespoon dried rose petals, to serve (optional)

1 tablespoon lime zest, to serve (optional)

Preheat the oven to 325°F and line an 8-inch square brownie pan with parchment paper or butter a nonstick saucepan (as shown).

Melt the butter in a saucepan until it darkens in color and smells nutty.

Mix together the sugar, cacao powder, flour, baking powder, and salt in a large bowl, then slowly pour in the melted butter, beating it in to blend. Add the vanilla extract, then beat in the eggs. Stir in the chia seeds until just combined, and then pour the batter into the prepared pan.

Bake for 20 minutes, or until a toothpick comes out with just a few moist crumbs attached and cracks form across the top. Let cool before removing from the pan, sprinkling with dried rose petals and lime zest (if using), and cutting into squares or slices.

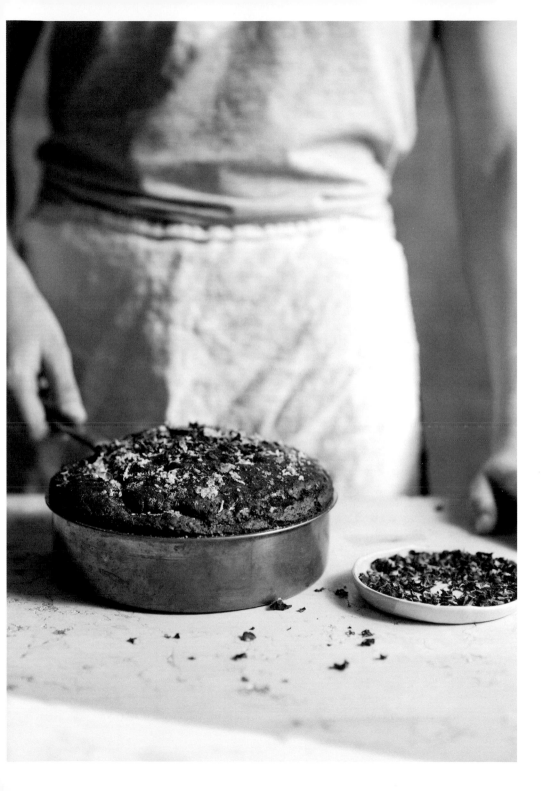

HOMEMADE CHOCOLATE BARS

This is an easy way to make homemade chocolate, which is just
about the perfect holiday or birthday gift. To make these bars, you
will need a silicone chocolate bar mold, available online or in baking
stores. Be creative with the toppings—what do you like?

¼ cup cacao butter

1 tablespoon coconut oil

3 tablespoons cacao powder

2 tablespoons agave syrup

1 teaspoon vanilla extract

pinch of sea salt

Topping options

dried edible flowers

Himalayan salt

freeze-dried raspberries

chopped nuts

cacao nibs

Melt the cacao butter and coconut oil in a bain-marie:
Set a heatproof bowl over a small saucepan of barely
simmering water, making sure the bottom of the
bowl doesn't touch the water. When it is completely
liquid, stir in the cacao powder, followed by the agave
syrup, vanilla, and salt. Stir until all the ingredients are
thoroughly combined and you have a silky texture.

Pour the mixture into your molds of choice and sprinkle
with your chosen toppings. Place in the freezer for
1 hour to set, then remove from the molds and wrap in
wax paper. Store in the refrigerator for up to 4 months.

BLACK SESAME SNAPS

These make a wonderful snack. You don't need to use black sesame seeds if you only have the white seeds on hand, although they look amazing. Sesame seeds are a rich source of healthy fats, which is why they work well as an energy snack.

1⅓ cups black sesame seeds

⅓ cup honey, plus 1 tablespoon

2 tablespoons coconut milk

sea salt

1¾ oz solid (100 percent) cacao chocolate

Preheat the oven to 350°F and grease and line a baking sheet with parchment paper.

Mix together the sesame seeds, honey, 1 tablespoon of the coconut milk, and a pinch of sea salt. Transfer the mixture to the lined baking sheet and flatten out with the back of a spoon, noting that it will spread a little more in the oven. Bake for 5–7 minutes. Let cool, then break into snack size pieces.

Meanwhile, melt the solid cacao chocolate in a bain-marie: Put into a heatproof bowl with the remaining tablespoon of coconut milk and set over a saucepan of barely simmering water, making sure the bottom of the bowl doesn't touch the water. Remove from the heat and stir through the remaining honey.

Dip the sesame snaps into the melted cacao and place on the now cool lined baking sheet. Cool the snaps in the refrigerator to solidify the chocolate, then transfer to an airtight container and keep for up to a week.

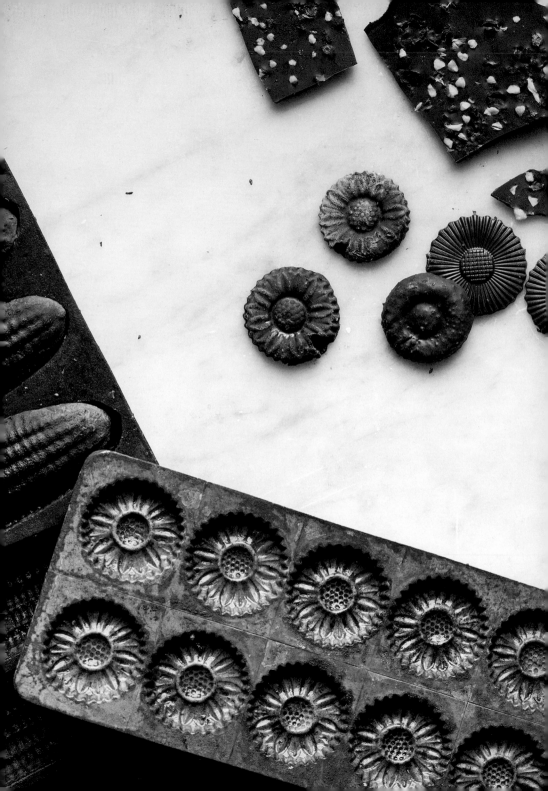

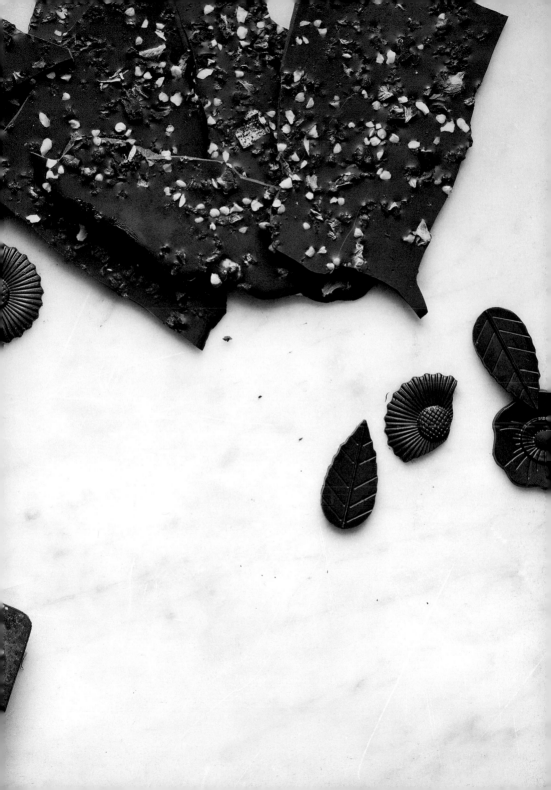

DEEP-FRIED CACAO RAVIOLI

Ravioli might not be the first thing that springs to mind
as a dessert, but the combination of orange zest, cacao,
creamy ricotta, and honey turn these pasta packages into
hard-to-resist bites.

3 eggs, beaten

2 cups "00" Italian flour or
all-purpose flour, plus extra
for dusting

1 tablespoon extra virgin olive oil

1 teaspoon sea salt

½ cup ricotta

zest of ½ orange

1 tablespoon cacao powder

1 egg white, beaten

vegetable oil, for frying

To serve

honeycomb, or honey

Greek-style yogurt

cranberries or raspberries

Mix the eggs, flour, extra virgin olive oil, and salt in a
large bowl with your hands or in the bowl of a food mixer
until a dough forms. Continue to knead by hand or with
the dough hook attachment of the mixer for about 10
minutes, until the dough is smooth and elastic. Wrap the
dough in plastic wrap and put into the refrigerator for
30 minutes.

Meanwhile, combine the ricotta, orange zest, and cacao
in a small bowl and set aside.

Lightly dust a pasta machine and cut your pasta dough
into four equal pieces. Starting at the widest setting, roll
the dough through the machine. Fold the pasta in half
and roll the dough through the same setting once again
before repeating at the next setting. Continue rolling
the dough until you get to the thinnest setting to create
four thin sheets of pasta.

Place teaspoonfuls of the ricotta mix at 2½-inch
intervals along the bottom edge of each sheet.

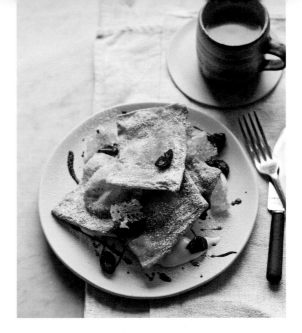

Brush the egg white around the ricotta and fold the top half over the bottom half, enclosing the ricotta. Cut the ravioli with a sharp knife or a serrated pastry cutter. You can chill the ravioli at this stage until ready to cook.

When you are ready to cook the ravioli, fill a saucepan with oil to about 2 inches deep and use a kitchen thermometer to heat the oil to 350°F. If you don't have a thermometer, you can test the oil by dropping in a small scrap of pasta dough; it should sizzle when it hits the oil. Add the ravioli, in batches, cooking them for 3 minutes, until they are a light golden color. Remove with a slotted spoon and drain on paper towels.

Serve with Greek-style yogurt, honeycomb, and cranberries or raspberries.

SERVES 6

◇◇◇◇◇◇

PANCAKES
WITH MELTED CACAO

This is a really simple crowd pleaser of a dessert or Sunday morning treat. When combined with the cacao chocolate, the butter works a little like cocoa butter to soften the bitterness. Similarly, the maple syrup adds a little natural sweetness.

2¾ cups chickpea (besan) flour

2 pinches of sea salt

coconut oil, for frying

To serve

butter

2¾ oz solid (100 percent) cacao chocolate, coarsely broken into pieces

maple syrup

ground cinnamon, chili flakes, or crushed pink peppercorns

sea salt

To make the pancakes, put the flour into a large bowl and stir through a good pinch of salt. Make a well in the middle and slowly pour in 1²/₃ cups water, whisking all the time, until you have a smooth batter. Set aside for at least 30 minutes at room temperature (even better, make the batter the night before).

To cook the pancakes, heat a little coconut oil in a nonstick skillet. When hot, ladle enough batter into the pan to make a pancake in a size of your choice. Cook for a couple of minutes, then flip over to cook for the same amount of time on the other side. Place on a hot serving plate and immediately add a pat of butter, a few pieces of chocolate, and a generous drizzle of maple syrup. Repeat with the remaining batter until it all has been used.

To serve, sprinkle cinnamon, chili flakes, or crushed pink peppercorns over the melting butter and cacao and finish with a few sea salt flakes.

SALAME DE CHOCOLATE

Similar to rocky road, *salame de chocolate* is popular in Portugal and is easy to make. We have added some dried cherries to the traditional recipe and replaced the plain cookies with gingersnaps.

¼ cup slivered almonds

¼ cup pistachios, chopped

1¾ sticks (¾ cup plus
    2 tablespoons) unsalted butter

⅓ cup coconut palm sugar or
    dark brown sugar

2 egg yolks

2 tablespoons cacao powder

1 cup semisweet chocolate chips

20 gingersnaps (about 5 oz),
    coarsely broken

⅓ cup dried cherries

1 tablespoon confectioners' sugar
    (optional)

Preheat the oven to 350°F.

Spread out the almonds and pistachios on a baking sheet and toast in the oven for about 7 minutes. Remove from the oven and transfer to a bowl to cool.

Melt the butter in a saucepan over low heat. Remove from the heat and stir in the coconut palm sugar, egg yolks, cacao powder, and chocolate chips. Return to low heat and stir continuously until all the ingredients are melted and combined to a smooth consistency.

Pour the chocolate mixture into the bowl with the toasted almonds and pistachios and mix thoroughly. Add the gingersnaps and cherries and stir to combine, then chill in the refrigerator for about 15 minutes.

Transfer the chilled chocolate dough to a sheet of wax paper and mold it into a cylinder shape. Roll the paper tightly around the dough and twist the ends, then roll the log on an even surface to create a smooth, salami-like shape. Chill for about 4 hours.

Remove from the refrigerator and unwrap the chocolate salami from the wax paper. Dust with confectioners' sugar, if using, and slice off pieces to serve. Wrap up again in the wax paper to store in the refrigerator for up to 7 days.

BRAZILIAN BRIGADEIRO

These traditional Brazilian sweets are simply cacao, butter, and condensed milk,
so they are definitely not a low-calorie treat, but you do need only one small
truffle to feel like you are indulging yourself!

3 tablespoons unsalted butter,
  plus extra for greasing
1⅓ cups sweetened condensed
  milk
pinch of sea salt
¼ cup cacao powder
1 teaspoon vanilla extract

To decorate
chopped pistachios
unsweetened dry coconut flakes
cacao powder
cacao nibs

Lightly grease a large plate.

Put the butter, condensed milk, salt, and cacao powder
into a heavy saucepan and place over medium heat.
Bring slowly to a boil, stirring constantly with a
wooden spoon. Reduce the heat to medium-low and
cook for 10–15 minutes, stirring constantly, until the
mixture is thick and shiny and starts to pull away from
the bottom of the pan.

Stir in the vanilla and vigorously mix again. Pour
the mixture onto the greased plate and chill in the
refrigerator for at least 2 hours.

Butter your hands and pinch off some of the dough to
make walnut-size balls. Put your coating ingredients
into small bowls and roll the balls in one of the bowls.
Place in mini paper liners or on a tray lined with
nonstick parchment paper.

Store in the refrigerator for up to 10 days.

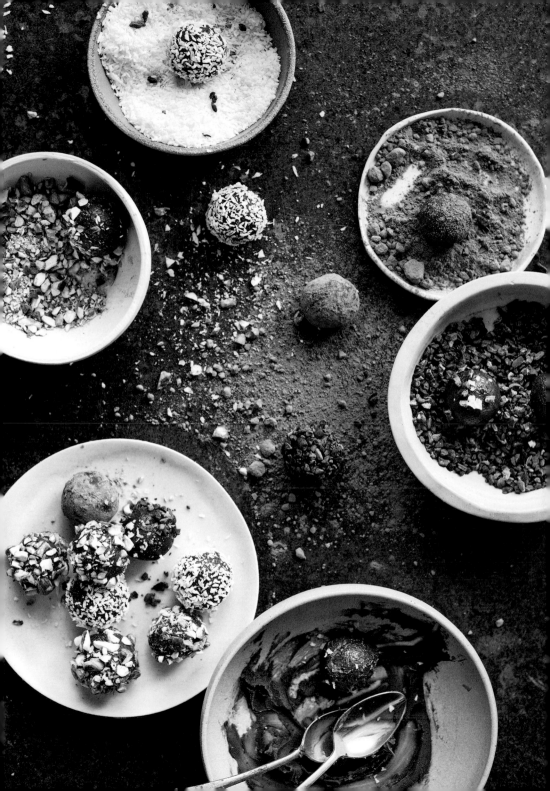

RAW CACAO
AND BLACK BEAN MOUSSE

Initially, you might think this recipe sounds pretty strange for a dessert—
black bean mousse? But we promise that you won't taste the beans; they simply
help create a fluffy consistency. Try them, you won't regret it! This is a dessert
with no guilt attached.

1⅓ cups drained and rinsed,
 canned black beans
½ teaspoon ground cinnamon
6 medjool dates, pitted
1 tablespoon coconut oil
1 tablespoon cashew nut butter
½ teaspoon vanilla extract
⅓ cup cashew nut milk
3½ oz solid (100 percent) cacao
 chocolate

In a food processor, blend together the black beans, cinnamon, dates, coconut oil, cashew nut butter, vanilla, and a little of the cashew nut milk until smooth.

Melt the chocolate in a bain-marie: Set a heatproof bowl with the remaining cashew nut milk over a saucepan of barely simmering water, making sure the bottom of the bowl doesn't touch the water. Whisk until smooth.

Let the chocolate mixture cool for a minute, then add to the ingredients in the food processor and blend until smooth.

Divide the mixture into individual glass jars or serving dishes and chill in the refrigerator for at least 3 hours before serving.

CACAO BUTTER FUDGE

This isn't a traditional fudge recipe, but it is smooth and chocolaty and, yes, you
could definitely mistake it for fudge.

¾ cup maple syrup

¾ cup chopped raw cacao butter

⅓ cup extra virgin coconut oil

½ cup coconut butter

1 teaspoon vanilla extract

pinch of sea salt

zest of 1 lime

Line a loaf pan with parchment paper.

Put the maple syrup into a small saucepan and bring to
a simmer over medium heat. Cook for a few minutes,
stirring occasionally, until it has reduced in volume by
about half. Set aside.

Meanwhile, put the cacao butter, coconut oil, and
coconut butter into a heatproof bowl and set it over
a small saucepan of simmering water, making sure
the bottom of the bowl doesn't touch the water. Melt
together until smooth. Remove from the heat and add
the thickened maple syrup, vanilla, and salt, stirring to
thoroughly combine.

Pour the mixture into the lined pan, sprinkle over lime
zest and chill in the refrigerator for 2–3 hours, until set.
Once set, turn out of the pan and cut into cubes.

Store in the refrigerator for up to 10 days.

CACAO BEET CAKE

Chocolate and beets are a match made in heaven, and this dark, almost flourless cake is an intense treat that actually contains loads of goodness.

8¾ oz solid (100 percent) cacao chocolate, coarsely chopped

3 extra-large eggs

1 cup packed light brown sugar

¾ cup all-purpose flour

½ teaspoon baking soda

1¼ teaspoons baking powder

pinch of sea salt

½ cup almond meal

1¾ cup shredded, peeled raw beets

⅓ cup sunflower oil

¼ cup avocado oil

For the topping

1 avocado

½ cup cacao powder

½ cup maple syrup

1 teaspoon rose water

Preheat the oven to 275°CF and grease an 8-inch loose-bottom cake pan. Line the bottom with parchment paper.

Melt the chocolate in a bain-marie: Put it into a heatproof bowl set over a small saucepan of simmering water, making sure the bottom of the bowl doesn't touch the water. Stir until smooth, then set aside to cool.

Using a handheld electric mixer, beat the eggs with the sugar in a large bowl until pale and fluffy. Fold in the flour, baking soda, baking powder, salt, cacao powder, and almond meal until thoroughly mixed together. Now fold in the beets, melted chocolate, and oils until evenly combined.

Pour the batter into the prepared pan and bake for 30 minutes in the center of the oven. Cover the cake with aluminum foil and return to the oven for another 30 minutes. Turn out of the pan and let cool on a wire rack.

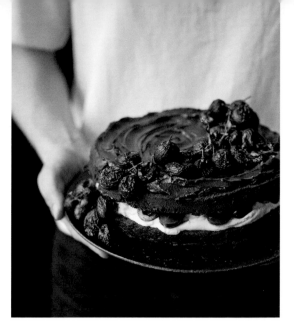

For the filling

2²/₃ cups black seedless grapes

1 tablespoon olive oil

1 cup Greek-style yogurt, strained
   through cheesecloth

To make the topping, put the avocado, cacao powder, maple syrup, and rose water into a food processor and process until smooth.

To roast the grapes for the filling, preheat the oven to 425°CF. Toss the grapes, still attached to the stems, in the olive oil and roast for about 30 minutes, until caramelized. Let cool, then remove half the grapes from the stems and slice in half, reserving the rest to garnish the cake.

Slice the cake into two disks. Spread the strained yogurt over the bottom half and add the halved grapes evenly. Top with the other half of the cake and spread over the cacao ganache topping. Arrange the roasted whole grapes still attached to the stems on the cake to serve.

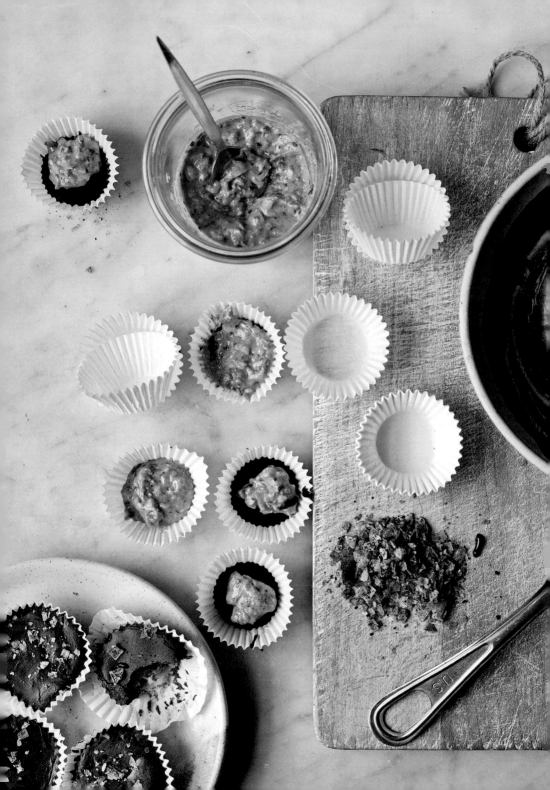

PEANUT BUTTER CACAO CUPS

These individual cups are a real treat, but the sweetness comes from honey or maple syrup instead of sugar, so they are an excellent alternative to most store-bought chocolates or sweet treats. They are also incredibly filling, so you won't be tempted to eat the whole batch.

½ cup coconut oil, melted

⅓ cup cacao powder

½ teaspoon vanilla extract

2 tablespoon raw honey or pure maple syrup

pinch of sea salt, plus extra for topping

raw peanut butter or almond butter (stir well and chill in the refrigerator ahead of time)

Mix together the coconut oil, cacao powder, vanilla, honey or maple syrup, and sea salt in a bowl. Pour a small amount of this chocolate mixture, about 2 teaspoons, into mini paper liners. Place them on a small tray and transfer to the freezer for 5 minutes to make the chocolate firm.

Remove the tray from the freezer and spoon a small dollop of peanut butter in the center of each cup. Add more of the chocolate mixture to each cup until filled to the top. Return to the freezer for another 5–10 minutes, until the chocolate has set solid. Sprinkle with a few sea salt flakes.

Store in the refrigerator for up to 10 days.

STICKY RICE PUDDING
WITH MANGO

This is a stove-top rice pudding to die for. If you are feeling more saintly than us,
swap the heavy cream for Greek-style yogurt.

¼ cup short-grain rice

½ cup coconut milk

1 tablespoon agave nectar or
   coconut syrup

zest of 1 orange

1 tablespoon cacao powder

1 vanilla bean, split lengthwise
   and seeds scraped a little

¼ cup heavy cream

zest of a lime

squeeze of lime

1 ripe mango, diced

cacao nibs, to serve

Put the rice, coconut milk, agave or coconut syrup,
orange zest, cacao powder, and vanilla bean (with seeds)
into a saucepan and bring to a boil over medium heat.
Reduce the heat and simmer for about 30 minutes, until
the rice is cooked, stirring often to prevent it from
sticking to the bottom of the pan. Remove from the heat
and let cool for a few minutes before stirring through
the cream.

Serve the rice pudding warm or chilled with the lime
zest and juice, mango, and cacao nibs.

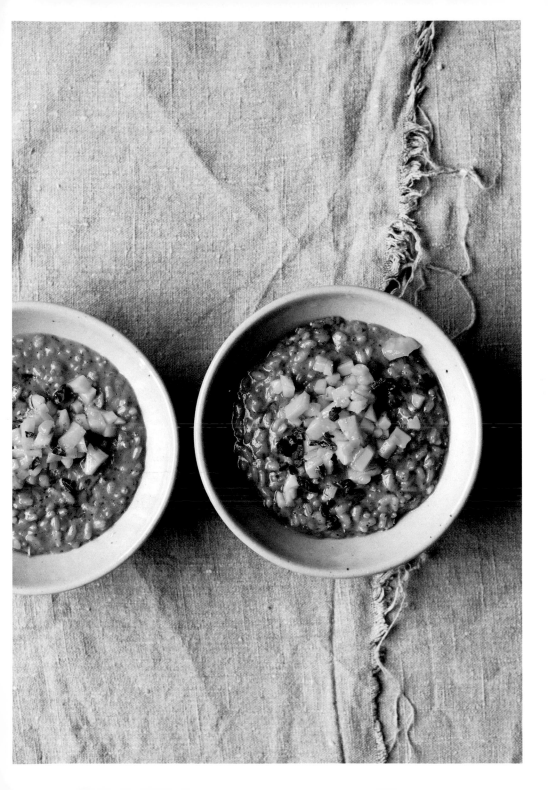

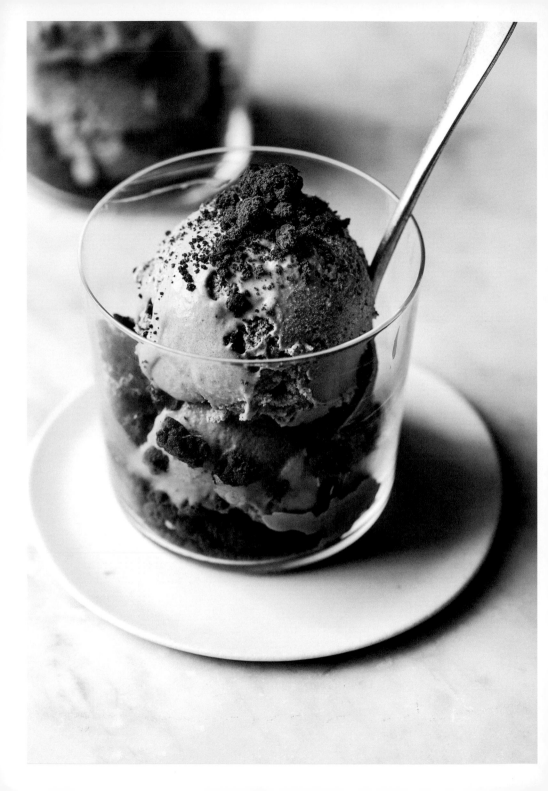

CACAO AND LEMONGRASS ICE CREAM

The lime leaves and lemongrass add a tart freshness alongside the dark cacao, while the chocolate soil adds the perfect crunch with a wonderful bitter edge.

---

2 cups whole milk

¾ cup superfine sugar

2 heaping tablespoons cacao powder

6 kaffir lime leaves, fresh or dried

1 lemongrass stalk, smashed

4 egg yolks

For the chocolate soil

¼ cup all-purpose flour

⅓ cup cacao powder

2 tablespoons coconut palm sugar or dark brown sugar

pinch sea salt

3 tablespoons unsalted butter, melted

Pour the milk into a saucepan, add half the superfine sugar, place over high heat, and bring just to a boil. Remove the pan from the heat.

In a bowl, make a paste with some of the hot sweet milk and cacao powder. Whisk it into the hot milk. Add the lime leaves and lemongrass stalk to the pan and let steep, covered with a lid, until the mixture is cold.

Using an electric whisk, beat the egg yolks with the remaining sugar until combined and creamy. On a low setting, slowly add the cooled milk (with the lemongrass and lime leaves removed). When completely combined, pour back into the pan and heat gently, stirring continuously, until thickened.

Chill for an hour, stirring occasionally, before churning for about 30 minutes to reach a soft serve consistency. If freezing, transfer to a suitable container and let soften for 15 minutes before serving.

For the chocolate soil, preheat the oven to 320°F and line a baking sheet with parchment paper. Mix the flour with the cacao powder, coconut sugar, and salt. Pour in the melted butter and mix. Spread out over the lined pan and bake for 15 minutes. Set aside and let cool before using.

BEAUTY

FACE MASK

Cacao is rich in antioxidants called flavonoids, which aren't just good for us to include in our daily diet, but are also great for the skin, stimulating circulation and smoothing fine lines. Antioxidants are essential anti-agers, fighting free radical damage and repairing skin cells. Cacao is also anti-inflammatory, so it can help to soothe redness and reduce skin blemishes. This simple face mask combines cacao with clay, which helps to draw out toxins and protect and nourish the skin with its rich mineral content.

---

1 tablespoon raw cacao powder
1 teaspoon bentonite clay powder
    (available online)
½ teaspoon avocado oil
diluted apple cider vinegar
    (1 tablespoon apple cider
    vinegar to ⅓ cup water)

Stir the cacao powder and bentonite clay powder together with a nonmetallic spoon. Mix in the oil, then add the diluted apple cider vinegar, one tablespoon at a time, until you reach a creamy, pastelike consistency.

Apply in a thick layer over cleansed skin, avoiding the eyes, and let soothe for 10 minutes.

Use an old facecloth to remove the mask, because it will stain. Simply soak it in lukewarm water, squeeze out the water, and hold it against your face to feel the warmth for a couple of seconds before gently wiping away the mask. Repeat until all the mask has been removed, then rinse your face with cool water and pat dry.

Apply a little facial oil or moisturizer.

BODY BUTTER

In warm climates, you might need to keep this body butter in the refrigerator to prevent it from melting. You can also reduce the amount of coconut oil in warm seasons and use 40 drops of a favorite essential oil as an alternative to the vanilla extract. When you use this body butter, it melts quickly on the skin and at first appears to be oily, but the oils are quickly absorbed and it is intensely moisturizing.

⅓ cup raw cacao butter
¼ cup coconut oil
1 teaspoon vanilla extract

Melt the cacao butter in a bain-marie: Put it into a heatproof bowl set over a saucepan of gently simmering water, making sure the bottom of the bowl doesn't touch the water. Stir in the coconut oil until the mixture is completely liquid.

Remove from the heat, stir in the vanilla extract (or essential oil), and let cool for about 10 minutes. Chill in the refrigerator for about 45 minutes, until the mixture begins to solidify (or about 10 minutes in the freezer). The mixture will change from a clear appearance to being opaque.

Use a handheld blender to beat the mixture. Let stand for 30 minutes, until it becomes fairly solid in texture, and work it into a cylinder shape. Use wax paper to wrap around the "butter" and smooth the shape. Transfer to an airtight container and keep for up to 4 months. You can slice off disks when you whant to use it.

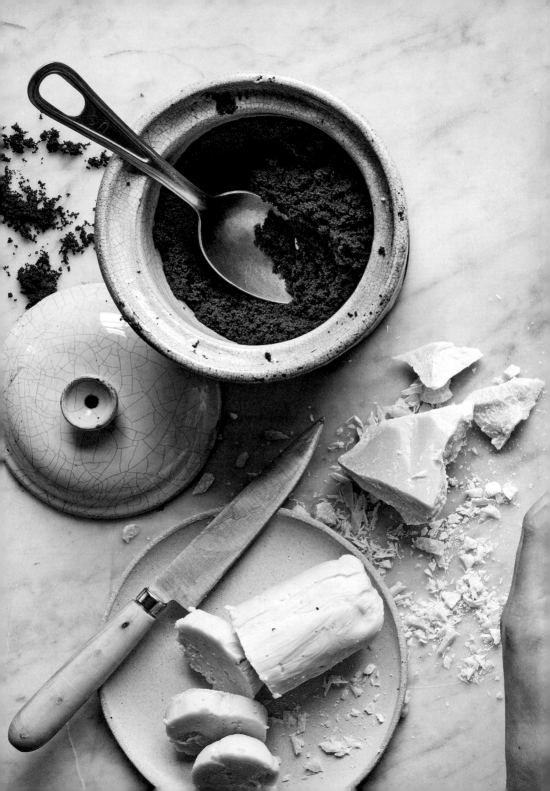

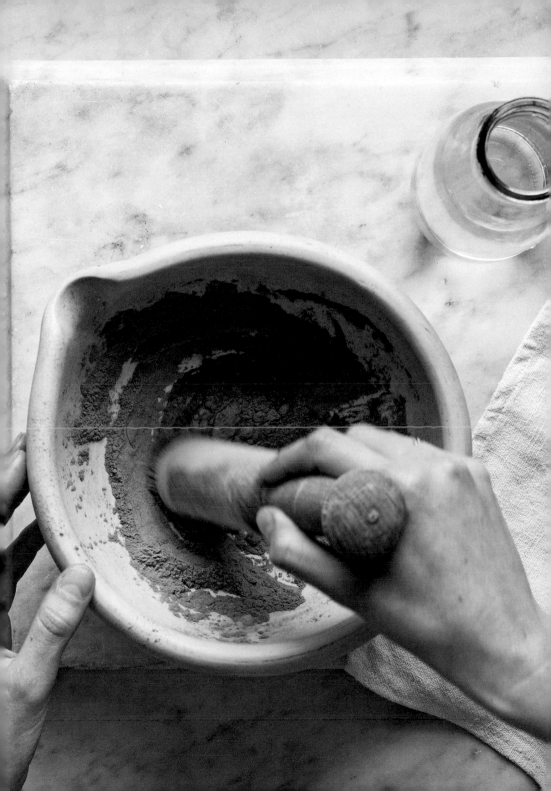

BODY SCRUB

This body scrub is a delicious way to exfoliate your skin with the grainy sugar and relieve dryness with the avocado oil and anti-inflammatory cacao. Natural body scrubs also make beautiful presents when presented in mason jars.

1 cup granulated sugar or coconut palm sugar

⅓ cup cacao powder

1 teaspoon vanilla extract

2 tablespoons avocado oil

Combine the sugar and cacao powder in a mixing bowl. Add the rest of the ingredients and mix until thoroughly combined. Transfer to a wide-rimmed airtight container.

To use in the shower, step aside from the water flow, scoop the scrub out of the jar, and apply to damp skin, paying attention to your feet and elbows. Rinse off in the shower.

FOOT CREAM

With its combination of essential oils, this foot cream will wake up
tired feet and moisturize and soothe away the day.

¼ cup shea butter

2 tablespoons raw cacao butter

20 drops of rosemary essential oil

20 drops of peppermint essential
oil

10 drops of lavender essential oil

10 drops of tea tree essential oil

Put the shea and cacao butters into a heatproof bowl
and set over a small saucepan of gently simmering
water, making sure the base of the bowl doesn't touch
the water. Melt until the mixture is completely liquid.

Let cool for 10 minutes, stir through the essential oils,
then cover the bowl and transfer to the freezer to chill
for 10–15 minutes, until solid but not too hard.

Using a handheld blender, mix until soft and whipped
in texture. Transfer to a wide-rim airtight jar.

To use, simply scoop out a small amount of cream and
indulge your feet.

CARDAMOM CACAO BATH MILK

Adding milk to a bath is a wonderful way to turn a bath into a soothing ritual,
and it's also really good for softening and renewing your skin. Both silk powder
and coconut milk powder are a little unusual but are available to purchase online.
Silk powder is used to create a softer texture.

---

2 tablespoons raw cacao butter

½ teaspoon silk powder

generous ½ cup coconut milk
    powder

1 tablespoon rose water

1 teaspoon ground cardamom

Combine the cacao butter, silk powder, half the coconut
milk powder, and the rose water in a small food processor
or spice mill and grind until fine. It will be a little pasty
to touch.

Scrape out into a bowl and add the remaining coconut
milk powder, mixing and breaking up any clumps
to make it as powdery as you can. Add the ground
cardamom and combine thoroughly. Transfer to an
airtight glass jar.

To use, add a generous sprinkle to a hot bath or foot
bath, swirling to dissolve in the water.

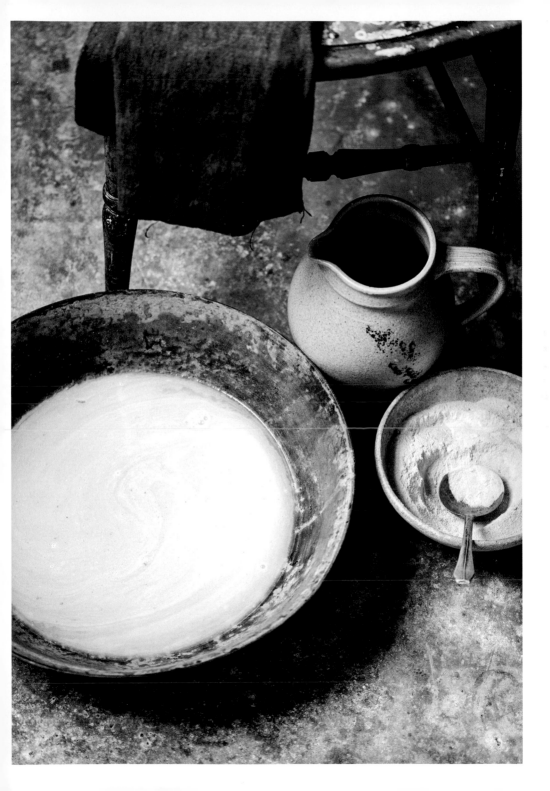

INDEX

◇◇◇◇◇◇

A

acai cacao smoothie 26
almond milk
    hot cacao 23
    overnight oatmeal 35
almonds
    cacao crusted cod 78
    Catalan chicken picada 80
    salame de chocolate 103
antioxidants 14
apricots
    protein breakfast bars 41
avocado
    avocado shrimp tortillas
        with blood orange cacao
        vinaigrette 71
    cacao beet cake 108–9
    cacao matcha smoothie 28
Aztec mythology 10

B

bacon
    beef short ribs with cacao
        and orange 86–87
banana
    acai cacao smoothie 26
    cacao matcha smoothie 28
    peanut butter chia 29
barbecue chicken 90
beans
    black bean and corn chili
        shakshuka 68
    homemade baked beans 49
    mackerel with cacao black
        beans 74–75
    raw cacao and black bean
        mousse 106
beauty recipes
    body butter 119
    body scrub 122
    cardamom cacao bath milk
        124
    face mask 118
    foot cream 123
    matcha face mask 120

beef
    beef short ribs with cacao
        and orange 86–87
    onglet with cacao
        butter 91
beet
    cacao beet cake 108–9
blueberries
    acai cacao smoothie 26
    granola 34
body butter 119
body scrub 122
bran muffins 38
Brazilian brigadeiro 104
bread
    burrata with clementine and
        cacao nibs 63
    Catalan chicken picada 80
    melted cheese sandwich and
        cacao relish 45
    Turkish eggs 46
brownies
    cacao chia pan brownie 94
buckwheat
    cacao crusted cod 78
    cauliflower soup with cacao
        buckwheat 54
burrata with clementine and
    cacao nibs 63
butter
    Brazilian brigadeiro 104
    Dublin Bay prawns with
        cacao butter 77
    onglet with cacao
        butter 91
    roasted cauliflower with
        cacao and paprika
        butter 60
butternut squash
    beef short ribs with cacao
        and orange 86–87
    black bean and corn chili
        shakshuka 68
    squash, cashew nut, and
        cacao soup 53

C

cacao 6–7
    cacao ceremony 12
    cooking with cacao 16
    health benefits 14–15
    hot cacao 23
    solid (100 percent) cacao
        chocolate 8
cacao butter 8
    cacao butter fudge 107
cacao nibs 8
    burrata with clementine and
        cacao nibs 63
    toasted cacao nibs 17
cacao powder 8
caffeine 15
calcium 14
cardamom cacao bath milk 124
cardamom roasted sweet
    potato with cacao and
    pomegranate molasses 64
Catalan chicken picada 80
cauliflower
    cauliflower soup with cacao
        buckwheat 54
    roasted cauliflower with
        cacao and paprika
        butter 60
cheese
    baby kale and quinoa salad
        with feta and lime cacao
        dressing 65
    cacao cheese straws with
        spiced yogurt 56
    deep-fried cacao ravioli
        100–1
    melted cheese sandwich and
        cacao relish 45
    lamb ragu with pappardelle
        88
cherries
    salame de chocolate 103
chia seeds
    cacao chia pan brownie 94
    peanut butter chia 29

chicken
    barbecue chicken 90
    Catalan chicken picada
      80
chili
    black bean and corn chili
      shakshuka 68
    Dublin Bay prawns with
      cacao butter 77
    pork belly with cacao glaze
      81
    squash, cashew nut, and
      cacao soup 53
    Turkish eggs 46
chocolate
    black sesame snaps 97
    cacao beet cake 108–9
    homemade chocolate bars
      96
    pancakes with melted cacao
      102
    raw cacao and black bean
      mousse 106
    salame de chocolate 103
clementines
    burrata with clementine and
      cacao nibs 63
cocoa 8
cod
    cacao crusted cod 78
corn
    black bean and corn chili
      shakshuka 68
    cacao crusted cod 78
cream
    cardamom roasted sweet
      potato with cacao and
      pomegranate molasses
      64
    sticky rice pudding with
      mango 112
criollo beans 6

D
dates
    protein breakfast bars 41
    raw cacao and black bean
      mousse 106
duck with cacao risotto 84–85
Dublin Bay prawns with cacao
    butter 77

E
eggs
    black bean and corn chili
      shakshuka 68
    cacao and lemongrass ice
      cream 115
    Turkish eggs 46

F
face mask 118
fiber 15
foot cream 123
forastero beans 6

G
ginger and cacao biscotti 39
granola 34
grapes
    cacao beet cake 108–9

H
homemade baked beans 49
homemade chocolate bars
    96

I
ice cream
    cacao and lemongrass ice
      cream 115
iron 14

K
kale
    baby kale and quinoa salad
      with feta and lime cacao
      dressing 65

L
lamb ragu with pappardelle
    88
lemongrass
    cacao and lemongrass ice
      cream 115
limes
    avocado shrimp tortillas
      with blood orange cacao
      vinaigrette 71
    baby kale and quinoa salad
      with feta and lime cacao
      dressing 65

M
mackerel with cacao black
    beans 74–75
mango
    sticky rice pudding with
      mango 112
maple syrup
    cacao beet cake 108–9
    cacao butter fudge 107
    oatmeal of the gods 32
    pancakes with melted cacao
      102
    peanut butter cacao cups
      111
    tonic 24
matcha
    cacao matcha smoothie 28
milk
    Brazilian brigadeiro 104
    cacao and lemongrass ice
      cream 115
mole 72
    octopus with mole 72–73
mood booster 15
MUFAs (monounsaturated
    fats) 15
mushrooms
    duck with cacao risotto
      84–85
mythology 10

N
nuts
    cacao Brazil nut butter
      42
    cacao nuts and seeds 57
    granola 34
    salame de chocolate 103
    squash, cashew nut, and
      cacao soup 53

O
oatmeal of the gods 32
oats
    granola 34
    oatmeal of the gods 32
    overnight oats 35
octopus with mole 72–73
onglet with cacao butter
    91

oranges
  avocado shrimp tortillas
    with blood orange cacao
    vinaigrette 71
  beef short ribs with cacao
    and orange 86–87
  deep-fried cacao ravioli
    100–1
  tonic 24

P
pancakes with melted cacao
  102
paprika
  roasted cauliflower with
    cacao and paprika
    butter 60
pasta
  deep-fried cacao ravioli
    100–1
  lamb ragu with pappardelle
    88
peanut butter cacao cups
  111
peanut butter chia 29
pistachios
  salame de chocolate 103
pomegranate molasses
  cardamom roasted sweet
    potato with cacao and
    pomegranate molasses
    64
pork belly with cacao glaze
  81
protein breakfast bars 41
pumpkin seeds
  cacao nuts and seeds 57
  granola 34
  protein breakfast bars 41

Q
quinoa
  baby kale and quinoa salad
    with feta and lime cacao
    dressing 65

R
raisins
  bran muffins 38
raw cacao and black bean
  mousse 106

rice
  duck with cacao risotto
    84–85
  sticky rice pudding with
    mango 112

S
salame de chocolate 103
sesame seeds
  black sesame snaps 97
shrimp
  avocado shrimp tortillas
    with blood orange cacao
    vinaigrette 71
spices
  barbecue chicken 90
  cacao cheese straws with
    spiced yogurt 56
  ginger and cacao biscotti
    39
  hot cacao 23
  oatmeal of the gods 32
spinach
  cacao matcha smoothie
    28
  melted cheese sandwich and
    cacao relish 45
squash, cashew nut, and cacao
  soup 53
sweet potatoes
  cardamom roasted sweet
    potato with cacao and
    pomegranate molasses
    64

T
tomatoes
  baby kale and quinoa salad
    with feta and lime cacao
    dressing 65
  black bean and corn chili
    shakshuka 68
  Catalan chicken picada 80
  melted cheese sandwich and
    cacao relish 45
  octopus with mole 72–73
tonic 24
tortillas
  avocado shrimp tortillas
    with blood orange cacao
    vinaigrette 71

trinitario beans 7
Turkish eggs 46

V
venison with cacao yogurt 83
vinaigrette
  avocado shrimp tortillas
    with blood orange cacao
    vinaigrette 71

W
wine
  mackerel with cacao black
    beans 74–75

Y
yogurt
  cacao beet cake 108–9
  cacao cheese straws with
    spiced yogurt 56
  peanut butter chia 29
  Turkish eggs 46
  venison with cacao yogurt
    83